P9-CDZ-782

BREAST

CANCER

THE
COMPLETE
GUIDE

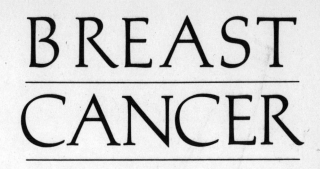

RC
280
.B8
H57
1996

BREAST
CANCER

THE
COMPLETE
GUIDE

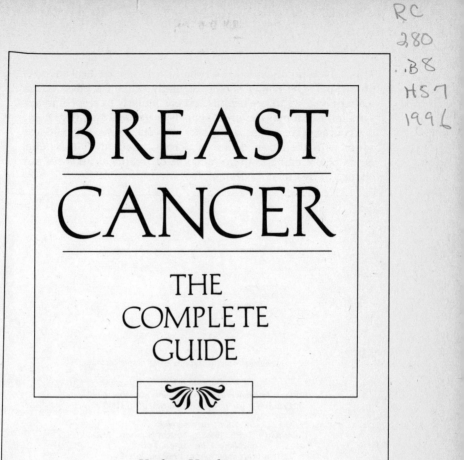

Yashar Hirshaut,
M.D., F.A.C.P.

and

Peter I. Pressman,
M.D., F.A.C.S.

Revised Edition

BANTAM BOOKS
New York • Toronto • London • Sydney • Auckland

WITHDRAWN
RARITAN VALLEY
COMMUNITY COLLEGE
LIBRARY

JUN 0 6 1997

This book is not intended as a substitute for the medical advice of physicians. The reader should regularly consult a physician in matters relating to her health, and particularly in respect to any symptoms that may require diagnosis or medical attention. As no one course of treatment is right for everyone, readers should also speak with their own doctor or doctors about their individual needs before embarking on a course of treatment and/or if any change in treatment is desired.

BREAST CANCER: THE COMPLETE GUIDE

A Bantam Book

Bantam hardcover edition published October 1992
Bantam trade paperback edition July 1993

All rights reserved.
Copyright © 1996, 1992 by Yashar Hirshaut, M.D.,
and Peter I. Pressman, M.D.
Illustrations copyright © 1992 by Jan Kays.
Book design by Robin Hoffmann, Brand X Studios.
Cover art copyright © 1996 by Belinda Huey.

No part of this book may be reproduced or transmitted
in any form or by any means, electronic or mechanical,
including photocopying, recording, or by any information
storage and retrieval system, without
permission in writing from the publisher.
For information address: Bantam Books.

Library of Congress Catalog Card Number 92-7576.

ISBN 0-553-37203-3

Published simultaneously in the United States and Canada

Bantam Books are published by Bantam Books, a division of
Bantam Doubleday Dell Publishing Group, Inc. Its trade-
mark, consisting of the words "Bantam Books" and the por-
trayal of a rooster, is Registered in U.S. Patent and Trademark
Office and in other countries. Marca Registrada. Bantam
Books, 1540 Broadway, New York, New York 10036.

PRINTED IN THE UNITED STATES OF AMERICA

FFG   0 9 8 7 6 5 4 3 2

*To our patients, for their trust
and friendship*

*To our wives and families,
for their support and encouragement
in the writing of this book*

We wish to thank Charlotte Mayerson
for her invaluable help in the organizing
and writing of this book

We are grateful to our colleagues
Doctors Nemetallah Ghossein, Bernard Kruger, Julie Mitnick,
Romulo Prudente, Richard Skolnik, and Robert A. Smith
for their kindness in reviewing
portions of this book

CONTENTS

Foreword by Amy S. Langer,
Executive Director, National Alliance of
Breast Cancer Organizations (NABCO)

BOOK I

FROM SUSPICION TO DIAGNOSIS

CONTENTS

BOOK II
TREATMENT

BOOK III
AFTER THE TREATMENT

BOOK IV
LIFE AFTER CANCER

FOREWORD

Amy S. Langer, Executive Director,
National Alliance of
Breast Cancer Organizations (NABCO)

Fate deals out some strange hands, as most people can confirm, but this seems particularly true in the case of a diagnosis of breast cancer. For a typical woman, the diagnosis is a jarring contrast to reality as she has been living it: feeling perfectly fine but finding, or being told about, a painless lump that may threaten her life.

This diagnosis—and the accompanying reality shift that inevitably follows—has become increasingly common. In fact, breast cancer is the most common form of cancer in women in the United States today. More frequently and at earlier ages, women are presented with a major medical problem that requires their levelheaded, informed participation to manage. At my organization, NABCO, we believe that the best resource for a woman facing breast cancer is information, and lots of it, that she can read, study, share with her family and friends, use as a basis for discussions with her physician, and rely upon as a way to feel back in control.

Amazingly, as recently as 1984 it was difficult to find good information about breast cancer treatment, whether as a confirmed or potential patient. Easy to find were experts who worked under the assumption that medical studies and journal articles were beyond the understanding of most women. These were the same physicians who found it appropriate to preface treatment recommendations with the phrase "If you were my wife," somehow never comforting or compelling.

Now, in 1996, women and their supporters can choose from a wide range of information and coping resources, *if* they know how to find them. A book can be the best first step, since it is available in stores and libraries everywhere and can be read, absorbed, and discussed according to a woman's own needs. *Breast Cancer: The Complete Guide* is such a resource, one that has become an invaluable addition to the field; and this new edition revises and extends the earlier work. The authors, both breast cancer experts, successfully combine accurate, up-to-date medical information with good, practical advice learned from women who have "been there." In an area where complex treatment options are constantly being refined, these two physicians present clear and concise outlines that provide a complete picture of choices for care. Very important, they assume that the reader is an intelligent, informed medical consumer who will work as an equal team member in managing the course of her care. And to their credit, they honestly acknowledge the difficult fact that in many treatment areas there is no one right answer.

The period from 1984 to 1996 is my personal window on the breast cancer landscape, since I was diagnosed with the disease in 1984, at the age of thirty. I had very lumpy breasts, and discovered a very early malignancy in a routine baseline mammogram that I scheduled, as casually as a dental checkup, on my gynecologist's recommendation. In the shock and fear that followed, I found that my best way of coping was to treat the diagnosis like a business problem, to shove it into the familiar analytical framework that I used at my Wall Street office every day. With steely resolve I set out to find out about the range of treatment options, not just here in New York, but also in Europe; who the real medical experts were who could care for me; what information resources were out there and how accurate and useful they were. I read endlessly, talked nonstop, hired and fired physicians. I cried, because it was a scary and lonely process. But at the end I made a truly informed decision that I felt fully confident about, and I knew what the next steps would be if the disease presented further problems or came back. This is the best kind of decision of all, and much easier to make today with a book like this one in hand.

Updating this foreword, first written for the book's debut in 1992, has offered the chance to reflect on the progress we have made in the fight against breast cancer. In the four years that have passed, scientists have made some astonishing discoveries and uncovered even more clues about how breast cancer starts, and therefore how we might soon be able to prevent and cure it. As was true in 1984 and in 1992, we still don't know for certain what causes this disease, and some women who do everything right—schedule routine mammograms, have annual clinical breast exams, and practice monthly breast self-examination—find breast cancer early, yet still die prematurely of their disease. However now, literally every month, researchers and clinicians publish advances in genetic mapping, diagnostic techniques, and treatment protocols that will rapidly translate into much better prospects for women with breast cancer and those at risk.

This acceleration of medical progress has largely been brought about by people concerned about breast cancer and women living with the disease. In 1992 the breast cancer advocacy movement was just getting off the ground. Since that time, millions of Americans have created the "politics" of breast cancer: they have marched and rallied, voiced their anger and frustration, and cast their votes based on attention given to breast cancer as a public health emergency. Men and women who would not continue to accept the legacy of breast cancer for their daughters and granddaughters have been the force behind a sixfold increase in the government's breast cancer research budget, and have inspired the launch of crucial private partnerships and crusades. As a direct result, the world of breast cancer will never be the same.

For many women reading this book, political action will seem very far away. Most readers will be women who feel at high risk for

FOREWORD

a diagnosis or who have already received one, since it is the practical truth that most of us don't research every possible health problem in advance. Very appropriately, the reader will focus on her own situation, considering what to do and how to cope.

I can advise you to take it step by step. Concentrate on the problems that are most pressing now, talk them through and decide, taking the next set of problems in turn. Know that you will come out of this, joining the nearly two million women alive in America today who have had breast cancer. Know that there are sources of help and support. Believe it or not, soon a whole day will pass when your diagnosis will not cross your mind once, when every twinge won't leave you panicked that it means more bad news.

When I first wrote these pages I was pregnant with my first baby, who turned out to be Henry. For me it was a time of great triumph and great hope. Now that same baby is three and a half, goes to school, is starting to read, and has just discovered knock-knock jokes. If in 1984 you had tried to reassure me that these future joys and comforts would be mine, I would never have believed you.

I can assure you that there is much to be learned and there are many personal victories ahead, even if you wish you could throw back this unwanted hand and be dealt another. Let this book, and your faith in yourself, be your guide.

New York, New York
January 1996

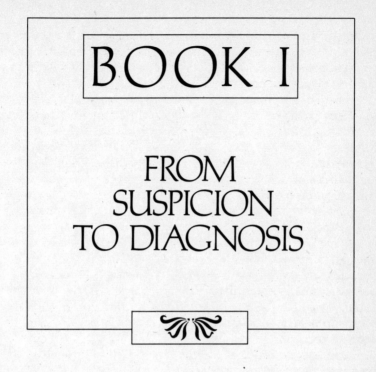

BOOK I

FROM SUSPICION TO DIAGNOSIS

1

HOW CAN A BOOK HELP ME?

The authors of this book are both physicians whose primary practices are in the field of breast cancer. Peter Pressman is a surgeon, Yashar Hirshaut an oncologist. We share a philosophy about staying involved in all the phases of treating our patients, and in that sense, we are both oncologists, one surgical, the other medical.

Both of us spend every day of our working lives with women who have breast cancer or fear that it lies before them. We have seen how they and their friends and families can sometimes be overwhelmed by this information, unclear as to how to proceed either in the practical matters or in the often devastating emotional ones.

The aim of this book is to provide you with a thorough, clear, step-by-step guide through the illness. More than that, we hope to act as "your brothers, the doctors," as people who care about you and want to share with you what we've learned from years of study and experience.

Why can't you get that kind of advice from your own physician? We certainly hope you can. But even the possibility of breast cancer poses problems so unusual that having an additional expert at your side may be of real help to you.

For example, if you've been told you have an appendicitis, even though it's an emergency, the course of treatment is pretty straightforward. You should try to find a competent, well-trained, and experienced surgeon who will do the procedure at a good hospital. But you don't have to worry about the physician's philosophy toward appendectomy. You don't, in general, have to worry about which type of surgery he'll perform. There are not several possible postoperative treatments to choose among.

More important, your survival chances after the removal of an unruptured appendix—unless there are unusual and unforeseen complications—are excellent. And unless you're a belly dancer or a bodybuilder, your concern about a small scar at the side of your abdomen is probably minimal. To put it another way, losing your appendix doesn't have much impact on your physical or social well-being, nor does it pose much of a threat to your self-image.

If, however, you've been told you may have breast cancer, you are facing all of those complexities—and more. It is our hope that this book will help women sort out such problems and approach them with as much confidence as possible.

As you may already have noticed, we are concentrating on breast cancer in women. We will not be addressing the illness in men, in whom it is rare, though the material on diagnosis and treatment would apply to them as well.

One other explanation: as a rule, we will use the first person singular "I" throughout the book because that seems most comfortable for us. In fact, sometimes one of us will be the basic expert in a chapter, sometimes the other, and in some sections the material will be the result of a pretty evenhanded sharing of expertise and experience.

The book is sprinkled with stories about women (anonymous, of course) whom we have known in our daily work. We have used these anecdotes to help us explain the conditions we are describing, and also because we think it may be useful to you to read about other women who have "been there," to hear what they felt and experienced, and how they coped. Much of our own insight into the illness has come from them.

The best understanding of breast cancer and its treatment will probably come from reading this book straight through. Doing that will also guide you, step by step, through any experience you may confront. If, however, you have a particular question to which you want an immediate answer, you can refer to the Contents or the Index and go right to the section that concerns you. There, if they are necessary, you will find cross-references to other pertinent material in the book.

Book I takes you from the time you first suspect a problem through the diagnosis of what it is. It helps you put into place the best possible personal and professional support system, including a team of doctors. It explains what may have gone wrong in your breast, whether it is a type of cancer or some other condition. In addition to diagnosis, Book I also covers pathology, and provides guidance in making the best preparations for treatment after you've found out what's wrong.

Book II has to do with prognosis—the probable course of the illness—and treatment: describing the procedures and the side effects of surgery, radiation, chemotherapy, and breast reconstruction.

Book III is a discussion of what happens after the initial course of treatment. It covers the appropriate medical follow-up as well as any recurrence of the illness. The last two chapters of this section describe what we know about the causes and prevention of breast cancer and the directions in which new research is pointing.

The final section, Book IV, relies heavily on the experiences of our patients in coping with the emotional impact of this disease, in understanding the reactions of others, and in the positive as well as the negative consequences of breast cancer that so many women have told us about.

The latest statistics, as of this writing, show that one out of nine women in the United States will develop breast cancer in her lifetime. There does seem to be a slow increase in the incidence of the disease. There are more new cases of breast cancer among women than of any other cancer.

That is not good news. Clearly, we have to find out what is going on and why. But the fact is, we know more about the disease every day. The cure rate is definitely increasing; though more women are now getting the disease, a larger percentage of them is surviving.

We now know how to treat breast cancer without the devastation of women's lives that was the norm only a decade ago. We also know that getting the right treatment from the right physicians can make all the difference. To help you do that is the purpose of this book.

CHAPTER

2

GETTING STARTED

W hen you or someone you care about has or is facing the possibility of breast cancer, it is natural to feel many bewildering and frightening emotions.

No one wants to get sick at all. Certainly no one wants to get cancer. And there are kinds of cancers that seem particularly terrible, not only because of their death-dealing potential, but because they or their treatment hits us "where we live." Breast cancer, for most women, is one of those diseases.

The possibility that you may have breast cancer is made even more stressful because it is an illness in which you are going to be called upon to make several decisions that don't necessarily arise in other situations. As we'll see later in this chapter, it's important that along with a carefully chosen team of physicians, you and the people in your personal support system take a very active role in the management of your case. Though that may feel a little intimidating right now, it can make a real difference in your welfare.

There are people who, when they are ill, take the attitude, "I'm going to find a good doctor and turn myself over to him. He knows better than I what should be done." Only to a certain extent is that a reasonable attitude in any medical situation. But breast cancer, with its many treatment possibilities, offers a special challenge to the patient.

WHAT DO I DO NOW?

For most of us, a serious threat to our health immediately takes center stage. Other concerns seem less important than they were before we learned of our illness. Though we may not articulate the thought, we understand that if we don't give first priority to taking care of the health crisis, there may not *be* any other concerns.

Even so, some women are so terrified of the thought of breast cancer that though they have found a lump or other abnormality in their breast, they suppress the knowledge, at least for a time. They may say to themselves, "That's nothing. I'm just imagining it," or "Next time I go to the doctor, I'll mention it," or "I've always had that. It's not worth worrying about."

Don't do this. We have seen too many women who became victims of their own fright and denial. Their illness, which would almost certainly have responded to treatment in its early stages, had so advanced by the time they sought help that it was too late.

So, the answer to the question "What do I do now?" is, first, get some perspective on what you are facing. Second, find good allies, the right doctors, to help you.

These are the concerns that women seem to worry about most:

Will I Survive?

Is the diagnosis of breast cancer a death sentence?

The answer isn't a simple "yes" or "no" but rather, in most instances, an optimistic "probably not, and certainly not immediately."

Those answers were not always available to us. A couple of

generations back, women did not talk about breast cancer and there was not nearly as much public discussion of the illness or the almost overwhelming coverage in newspapers and magazines, on radio and television, as occurs today. Self-examination was seldom done, and even when women did notice a small lump, they may have postponed taking any action out of a combination of ignorance and fear. Therefore, by the time they got to the doctor, they tended to be in later stages of the disease, and that very adversely affected their chances of beating it.

Moreover, in the past, the medical profession was much less effective in dealing with the illness than it is now. The prevailing treatments were, in general, less successful, more disfiguring, and more seriously disruptive of the quality of the patient's life. Surgery was much more extensive, chemotherapy and radiation techniques were less refined, and we did not have as much experience with their use, their results, and their side effects as we now do.

What Is Today's Success Rate?

To understand the changes that have taken place, bear in mind that a five-year length of time is often used to express the success rate. And though we'll get into the stages of cancer (see pages 40–41), for the purposes of this comparison it is enough to say that generally speaking, cancers are mainly classified by how far they have spread. With those factors in mind, it is encouraging to see how much progress we have made:

Between 1960 and 1964, the five-year survival rate for all stages of breast cancer was 64 percent. For local cancers, it was 84 percent. For cancers that had spread to lymph nodes near the affected breast, the rate was 54 percent. Where the cancer had spread to a distant site, only 7 percent of the affected women survived.

From 1979 to 1984, the five-year survival rate for all stages was 75 percent; for local cancers, 90 percent; for those that had spread to nearby lymph nodes, 69 percent; and for distant cancer, 10 percent.

The most recent five-year figures show an overall survival of 83 percent and parallel improvements in the other stages. For local cancers it is 96 percent; for those involving the regional lymph nodes, 75 percent; and for distant cancer, 20 percent.

So, many more women are surviving. That doesn't mean that

anyone can tell you definitively, without any doubt, that you are not going to be on the wrong side of the statistics. It does mean that your chances of conquering this condition are generally good.

Will I Be Disfigured?

Actually the question is often phrased more dramatically: many women use the word *mutilated*. "Will I be mutilated?" The answer to that is a lot easier. It's a clear and unequivocal "no."

In Chapter Seven, we will discuss in detail the various types of surgery for breast cancer. The relevant thing to say now, however, is that what women quite rightly dread most—the disfiguring **radical mastectomy,** in which the entire breast and a lot of the surrounding tissue and musculature are removed—is rarely needed anymore.

The **modified radical mastectomy** removes the breast but leaves the muscles intact. The result is much less damage to the body and a much better situation for breast reconstruction.

Many women now are treated with what is commonly called a **lumpectomy,** a surgical procedure that is technically referred to as a **wide excision.** In this technique for saving the breast, only the cancer, some surrounding tissue, and the nearby lymph nodes are removed. The remainder of the breast is then treated with radiation. These procedures will be discussed thoroughly in Chapters Seven and Eight.

Most important to this question of disfigurement is breast reconstruction. We will go into this subject in detail in Chapter Eleven, but it is helpful to realize that the techniques the plastic surgeons employ have been so refined in the past few years that after mastectomy, the breast can be reconstructed and a sense of wholeness almost completely restored. Most of my patients who have undergone reconstruction are pleased and relieved at the results.

The Question of Sex

Because women themselves consider their breasts to be a central part of their sexuality, as well as because of the frequent emphasis on the breast in the media and in art, many of them fear that breast cancer means an end to their sexuality—that they will no longer be attractive, or ever again enjoy sexual experience.

Let's begin with what I think is the common happy ending to this part of the story: there is no doubt that women and their sex partners may have complex issues to work out after breast cancer treatment. But from what I have seen in my practice, breast cancer seldom has long-term or disastrous consequences on the personal lives of my patients. There is a period of adjustment, but it's my impression that it isn't very long and that most couples put their fears behind them and reestablish satisfying and loving relations.

Many single women who are not in a relationship at the time of their illness have great fear—even a sad certainty—that a "new" person will not want to take on as awkward a situation as this. They may worry that they won't be attractive to someone who has not lived through this experience with them. Again, though this evidence can't be statistical, I hear wonderful stories of strong and happy relationships built after breast cancer.

In fact, though it may be hard for you to imagine now, women often find that this experience takes its place in their history just as other difficult life experiences do. They surely would not have chosen it, but having had breast cancer has by no means ruined their lives.

Here's what one woman, now in her late forties, had to say at her five-year checkup:

"I had a mastectomy and at first I was in pretty bad emotional condition. Reconstruction wasn't advised at the time and I'm not sure I would have wanted to go through more surgery anyhow. I didn't have a man in my life at the time and I thought to myself, Okay, kid, you better fill up your life with other things because romance is out from now on. Well, then I met Michael and I have to tell you I was shaking like a leaf the first time he even stood close to me because I was afraid he'd feel how my breast was gone and be really repelled. But that's not the way it turned out at all. In fact, when I told him, I think it opened him up to a lot of tenderness that was good for both of us and that's stayed on in our relationship."

Another woman, trying to decide with her husband and her doctor what course of treatment was best for her, heard her husband ask incredulously, "What makes you think the only place you're sexy is in your right breast?"

11

A third patient who was treated with only the removal of the cancerous lump and radiation now says that aside from a thin scar, her appearance has hardly changed.

Indeed, there are so many happy endings after breast reconstruction that it's hard to select among them.

The sum of these experiences? The majority of women who survive breast cancer make a good adjustment to any changes in their bodies that result from the illness or its treatment.

Dealing with Your Emotions

I had a patient in the office recently to whom I had to explain that the small lump on her breast was indeed cancer. For the rest of the visit she shut out all the reassurances I could truthfully give her, as well as all the conversation we needed to have about treatment. "Am I going to die?" she kept asking. "Promise me that I'm not going to die."

No one can do that, as much as I wished I could. Yet this woman's fear is perfectly understandable. It is perfectly natural. It's a fear that everyone in these circumstances experiences. But to get the best treatment possible, to put together the best team of doctors, services, and loving support, you can't panic and let your fright overwhelm you.

"Easy for you to say" may be your reaction to that statement. But, in reality, most women find that after the first shock of the threat of breast cancer, their own desire to survive soon pushes to the forefront. It overcomes any initial paralysis they may experience. They go ahead with what needs to be done to find expert help and to otherwise take care of themselves. (That patient I was describing came back a few days later, having absorbed the shock and far more ready to deal with her problem.)

Use whatever resources you can muster to support yourself emotionally. Talk to your husband or partner, to trusted family members, or to friends. Think about earlier challenges in your life and how you overcame them. Deep breathing exercises, meditation, and physical activity can be useful for some people during these first worrisome and uncertain days. That is especially true if you normally use such techniques for relaxation.

But, whether or not you do these things, it seems to me that you'll get the most comfort and confidence when you begin to understand that though you are confronting a new and frightening adversary:

- You are not alone.
- There are competent and experienced specialists who can help you.
- Other people are beating this enemy every day.

There's more to take comfort from in what we've learned thus far:

- You are almost certainly not facing immediate death.
- You will almost certainly not be disfigured.
- You are almost certainly not going to be shut off from the physical side of your life.

A Personal Support System

Put out of your mind any idea that you should "keep a stiff upper lip" or suppress your anxiety. Don't do that. Talk as much as you need to, to whoever will be the most helpful. That may or may not be your husband or partner. If the person who is closest to you is likely to panic at the thought that you have breast cancer, or has a completely different approach to illness than you do, turn to a friend or a close relative to act as your sounding board. Or take into your confidence another woman who has had breast cancer in recent years. Don't use these people *instead* of a doctor: use them as companions on this journey you're setting out on.

Ask one of the people you most trust to act as your personal advocate in the period ahead. See if that friend, or relative, or husband or partner, can accompany you to your medical appointments when you feel you need support or when you will be making treatment decisions. You may not want this personal ombudsman to take over for you, but it will be helpful if he or she keeps up with your case, knows your physicians, and understands you as a person. (For more detailed information on the use of a personal advocate, see page 95.)

The emotional concerns we've been discussing are shared by most women who face the prospect of breast cancer. The first practical problem they encounter is finding a doctor. That is the task we'll consider next.

FINDING A DOCTOR

Why do you have to find one? A doctor may have been the one who first felt the lump in your breast or saw something suspicious on a mammogram. If you found a lump yourself, you may have gone to your own physician or to someone at a group practice. Isn't the doctor already found by now?

Maybe, but not necessarily. Probably, to get the very best diagnosis and care possible, you should look beyond this first person you've seen, even though you may decide in the end that she is the best person to treat you. No matter where you live, no matter what your experience with medical problems, no matter what access to specialists and medical centers you've had up to now—you want to find the very best physicians possible for each aspect of your diagnosis, treatment, and follow-up. That search for a team of doctors—usually beginning with a surgeon—is what you and the people who are supporting you must now undertake. And if you consider the factors below, one by one, the task can be accomplished without too much difficulty and your choices will fall into place.

What Kinds of Doctors Treat Breast Cancer?

The place most people start this search is at the office of their *gynecologist* or their *family doctor*, who is sometimes an internist, a specialist in internal medicine.

You will have to ask yourself now whether you feel comfortable with the advice of this physician whom, up until now, you may have consulted only for fairly routine matters. Certainly you should consider the cancer specialist to whom she refers you, but

14

you should also feel free to do a careful search of your own to be sure you are getting the best advice and care.

If, in other family health crises, you were pleased with your physician's referrals, you can proceed more confidently. Your doctor has probably already sent patients to this breast cancer specialist and has had a chance to see favorable results. If your own physician is a caring and intelligent human being, there's a good chance she will at least get you started on the right track.

Unless your illness is already in an extremely advanced stage, it is almost certainly to a *surgeon* that you will be sent next for the purpose of diagnosis. Why is that? Isn't a surgeon most likely to want to "cut"? As you will see in Chapter Four, an essential early step in finding out what's wrong is often a biopsy—and a biopsy is surgery. It is a small operation, but a surgeon is best suited to perform it, not only because of his surgical skill, but because he has unique training that makes his opinion at both the diagnostic stage and the treatment stage invaluable.

Here's a helpful analogy: Trying to accurately assess a small mass that is deep in the breast is like trying to feel a pea hidden behind the thick folds of a curtain. Unless you draw the curtain aside, you can't be sure that something is really there, much less what exactly it is. A good breast surgeon, because he has so much experience, is probably better at feeling what is behind the curtain than most other physicians. And he is the only one who, if it is necessary, should draw the curtain open, that is, perform the biopsy.

The surgeons who specialize in breast cancer have board certification in general surgery. They may have taken special training in breast surgery and they have certainly devoted their practices primarily to this disorder.

An important member of the diagnostic team is the *radiologist*, a specialist who has been trained and certified in the use of X rays and other forms of imaging that are used to look inside the body. This specialist has become an extremely important player in the diagnosis process, as we will see in Chapter Four. That is in part because of recent dramatic improvements in mammography, the X-ray procedure that produces "pictures" of the breast called mammograms. Since mammograms are now routinely used for preventive as well as diagnostic purposes, and since the results are now so refined, it is very important to consult a particularly expert mammographer. Excellence in performing the examination and in interpreting its results is a very special skill not shared by all those who do this procedure.

The *radiotherapist* uses radiation after a lumpectomy is performed and sometimes following a mastectomy. Radiation therapy may also be used locally to control advanced disease. The role of such treatment will be explored in detail in Chapter Eight. (The radiotherapist is usually not involved in the diagnostic process.) Since breast tissue is extremely sensitive to damage by radiation, it is crucial to find competent and experienced practitioners who have at their disposal the best (and usually, unfortunately, most expensive) equipment possible for the planning and delivery of radiation treatment.

The medical *oncologist* generally sees breast cancer patients after the diagnosis and, usually, after any necessary surgery that follows. Medical oncologists are internists who specialize in the diagnosis and treatment of cancer. They most commonly use systemic therapy; that is, hormone therapy and chemotherapy, which act throughout the body in the prevention of the recurrence of the disease as well as in long-term care. Briefly, chemotherapy is the use of special drugs that have a specific destructive effect on cancerous tissue. The hormones used in treatment cause tumor shrinkage. (See Chapter Ten.) If a patient comes for treatment in a very advanced stage of breast cancer, the judgment may be made that surgery should not be used. (See page 129.) In that case, the oncologist will treat the patient from the start. (I have in my own practice many women who came to me with advanced cancer but who, nevertheless, have done well. One woman came to my office eighteen years ago with a cancer so extensive that there seemed no reason to subject her to useless surgery. She has had a course of medical therapy and is not only still alive, but seems fine.)

A *plastic surgeon* repairs skin and tissue. After a mastectomy, he may be called upon to reconstruct a treated breast. In Chapter Eleven, we will explore the techniques of the surgeons who do breast reconstruction. Their results are strikingly better than they were only a few years ago.

Who's in Charge?

You are in charge, in the sense that you will have to get enough information to be able to put together the team of specialists that is required for the best treatment of breast cancer. You should choose the best person you can find in each specialty. Who becomes the leader of the team depends on the nature of the illness, which doctor you need to see most frequently, who knows you best, and who is willing to act as leader. Ideally, the treatment of breast cancer is a cooperative effort with the command shifting as the need arises.

It is usually the surgeon who, at least initially, is the leader. It is he who must perform the biopsy. Furthermore, as we will explore when we discuss the treatment of cancer in Book II, in most cases the other treatments of breast cancer are used to supplement the effects of surgery. Nevertheless, the radiologist, the radiotherapist, the oncologist, the plastic surgeon, and the family doctor or gynecologist all play crucial roles, and each of these team members should be the very best physician available. What follows are guidelines to help you judge what "the very best" is, and then how to find it.

THE PERSONAL CHARACTERISTICS OF THE PHYSICIAN

The Doctor as Advocate

I have to start by explaining my own attitudes and biases. When I look around me, I see two different kinds of physicians. There are those who view themselves as objective professionals, very much like judges. Their attitude is impartial; the patient and the cancer stand before them at the bar as equals. Such doctors are at great pains to explain to cancer patients the "reality" of the dangers of the disease and the difficulties in fighting it. They are certainly pleased if the patient "wins," and they certainly take appropriate action in the treatment to try to achieve this end. But

17

they don't seem to be passionately on the patient's side, a feisty adversary to the cancer.

Then there is the defense attorney, the man or woman who gets in there—the tougher the case, the bigger the challenge—and fights for the client. That is the kind of doctor we all want: one who will not be intimidated by a grave illness, but who will fight it with all the vigor, skills, and techniques that can be mustered. Find that kind of doctor and you have a better chance to win your case.

The Involved Healer

There is another, subtler question I want to get into and that is to define for myself as a doctor how to be caring of my patients and yet not be overwhelmed by my sympathy. Like anybody else, when a doctor is overwhelmed, he's not in very good shape to make the best decisions.

I see my patients as individuals I care about and I want them to understand that. On the other hand, I want to be able to bring to their illness the kind of objectivity that good diagnosis and treatment require. To draw that fine line takes most doctors a long time to learn.

Once, many years ago, I was on my way home after a full day of tension and tragedy. In particular, one of my patients was doing very poorly, and I was lamenting the fates that had put her in such a position. And then I had an insight that has been a great help to me since then. I saw clearly that my role as a physician is not to lament but to find a way out—to look at the situation as it presents itself and to focus on finding constructive opportunities to make it better. It would not be helpful to the patient if I allowed myself to be paralyzed by anxiety. The patient needs a strong advocate, but one who can take an objective view of what is wrong, and then, with a cool head, develop a strategy for overcoming it.

This does not mean your doctor should not be closely involved. It's very important to find a physician with whom you can have a personal relationship, to whom you can give your confidence and from whom you feel a warm concern. Many doctors shun such a relationship. They try to stay emotionally detached. It's easy to understand why: they build a wall to protect themselves from getting hurt if the patient does not do well. But though this is not their intention, by reducing their vulnerability it seems to me they are also reducing their commitment. When the chips are down, such doctors may not fight as hard as they could. They may give up earlier than someone who has permitted himself to develop a warm, caring relationship with the patient.

And that is what you should look for: a doctor who will fight for you like a close friend. Avoid physicians who you think will insist on keeping their distance.

Patience

When you first meet a doctor you are considering, make sure that she is patient in hearing your story and evaluating your condition. It is up to the doctor to establish the kind of atmosphere that allows you to feel that you are getting all the time you need.

Some medical offices are so busy and the consulting rooms so tense that you feel you are being rushed, and that the doctor is anxious to get you moving through her "assembly line." If that is the feeling you get, trust it and look for someone else. Patience, the virtue our mothers talked about, is essential in a doctor who deals with breast cancer.

On the other hand, capable doctors are in demand and their waiting rooms are often crowded. I wish I could say that women never have to wait in my office, but they often do. We try to schedule enough time for each patient, but emergencies arise, or somebody needs an especially long and painstaking explanation of her situation or extra time for comfort and reassurance. It can be difficult to balance giving the person before you all the time she needs, and worrying about the patients you know are anxiously waiting outside.

Some of my patients handle the problem by calling ahead, before they leave for their appointment, to ask how we are doing, whether they should come right in or perhaps wait a half hour or so until the office traffic has eased.

19

Thoroughness

This quality is closely related to patience. It takes a fair amount of time during the first visit to take a patient's history and to give her a complete physical examination. If the doctor isn't thorough, it is almost certain that important details will be missed. Note whether the physician gives you a chance to tell her everything that has happened since you discovered a lump or were told that your mammogram was suspicious.

She should also take a full history of past medical problems, allergies, drugs you take, and all relevant family and social details. These should include questions such as: When did you begin to menstruate? What was the date of your last period? How many pregnancies have you had? How many children? How old were you when you had your first child? Does anyone in your family have cancer? Breast cancer? Your mother? Grandmother? Sisters? Cousins?

Watch to see whether the doctor takes her time during the physical examination. Does she examine both breasts? Does she carefully review the mammogram and any other test results you brought with you? Pay attention to these details and others like them to make sure that you are putting yourself in the hands of a meticulous person.

Careful Explanations

A good physician will encourage you to ask questions and will answer you thoughtfully and understandably. She will carefully explain to you the available options in your treatment and will ask what your feelings are about them. If a physician uses medical or technical terms that are not familiar to you, ask for a "translation" immediately. Do you understand what is wrong? What tests are needed? What treatment is planned? What alternative treatments may be available?

It is probably a good idea to bring someone with you to any early, exploratory appointments. Your companion can help you evaluate how the meeting went, and you will have someone to act as a sounding board in your later consideration of whether this particular doctor is the right person for you.

Your personal advocate can also help you remember the questions you should be asking as well as the answers the physician gives to them. In that regard, it's a very good idea to take with you to the doctor's office a small pad on which you've written your questions and can record her answers. Even if you ordinarily have a good memory, you may find that under stress you "lose" some information you need.

You should not feel any embarrassment about asking questions, consulting your notes, or writing down what the doctor says. More and more patients follow this procedure and find it very helpful.

Your Own Decision

It is essential that you feel comfortable with the doctor who will be in charge of your care. It is equally important, as we will see on page 27, that you be convinced that the particular approach to treatment that is being suggested is right for you.

These considerations are primary. If you are uncertain about any of them, you have every right to look further. This is much more important than worrying about hurting a doctor's feelings, or being embarrassed about asking for your X rays or records to take to another physician.

No one wants to be discourteous, and it's pretty safe to assume good intentions all around. But you have an absolute obligation to take the best care of yourself you can. That may mean "shopping around" and getting other opinions. It may mean insisting upon the release of the reports of the tests and diagnoses you have received (and paid for), taking your time in making decisions, and, if you like, having someone with you to consult with you and the physician.

Take Your Time

Don't feel rushed to make a decision about a doctor. Breast cancer should be treated as soon as possible, but that does not mean within a day or two and it certainly doesn't mean that speed is more important than making sound decisions.

The least satisfactory visits in my practice occur when a colleague calls and says, "There's a woman sitting across the desk from me whom I've known for years. She found a lump in her breast this morning and I want you to see her right away." If I examine that woman immediately, tell her she probably has cancer, and outline a proposed plan of treatment, it's likely to be a disaster. Here is a person who woke up that morning, presumably healthy, and suddenly her world has caved in. There's someone talking to her about the loss of her breast or how to conserve it. She's had no time to talk with her family or friends, to find out whom she really wants to consult with, or even to think about the questions she should be asking.

The first hours after you've been told that you may have breast cancer are bound to be upsetting. Anybody would feel, in those circumstances, as if the world had turned upside down. Give yourself time to talk to your family and friends and to compose yourself. Take your time. Tell any doctor who may be urging great haste upon you that you'd rather go home now and that you'll call him tomorrow or the next day. You may decide, in the end, to go to the specialist he's recommending, but you'll get a lot more out of that relationship if you haven't hurtled into it.

Searching for a Doctor

What is the best procedure to follow in finding these specialists? Even if the first doctor you see is someone you've known for years and whose good judgment has been proven to you repeatedly, give the matter some thought. Consider whether or not you want to shop around. You are not "stuck" with the doctor who finds the lump, or the first doctor you consult. You do not have to choose or stay with the specialist to whom you've been referred.

In practical terms, that means that if your gynecologist or family physician has found a lump in a routine examination, you may want to consult the breast specialists with whom he usually deals—or you may not. If you yourself have found the lump, you may want to go to your family doctor and have him manage your case—or you may not. If you go for an annual mammogram, you may want the results reported to the group practice you belong to—or you may not.

You should not prolong the search for a doctor as a way of avoiding timely action, nor should you keep "shopping" to the point of making yourself anxious and confusing the issue. But most insurance policies pay for—or even require—consultation at this point, so do get a second or even a third opinion until you like the physician you're dealing with and feel comfortable with her experience, training, hospital affiliation, and general approach to your particular situation. (We will discuss each of these factors later in this chapter.) You may get conflicting opinions you will have to choose among. But, until you feel comfortable with a particular plan of treatment, and confident in the abilities of each physician on the team, leave yourself open to other options.

"Network"

How do you find a good cancer specialist? Try to investigate the problem through a variety of sources. Talk to friends, relatives, and colleagues about finding a doctor. You'll be amazed at how many people have had firsthand experience either as patients themselves or with people close to them.

Keep a list of those doctors women liked and those they didn't. Pretty soon you'll notice that one or two names keep cropping up on the "good" side of your list. Get a sense from the people who mentioned them of what those physicians are like, their hospital affiliation, and their general approach to the illness. Use these names to start your quest.

Breast cancer is, unfortunately, common enough in most cities that there are doctors, particularly surgeons, who treat only that condition. They are, obviously, experienced in most of its aspects. Experience is a valuable asset.

If you live in an area where there are no breast specialists, you should consider whether it is feasible to consult one in a nearby city. Even if, in the long run, you are going to have to rely on ongoing treatment from a doctor in your own area, I'd suggest that at the time of diagnosis, and of any surgery, you try to consult with such a breast cancer specialist.

Other Ways to Search

What other steps can you take to find a good doctor?

- The National Alliance of Breast Cancer Organizations (NABCO) has compiled an excellent list of services and materials relevant to breast cancer. Their latest compilation of local support organizations can be found in the appendix of this book. Call the group closest to where you live for leads on finding a physician.
- Consult the telephone book or ask your county health department if there is a breast cancer hotline available in your area. Call the hotline for information about physicians in your community.
- The National Cancer Institute's (NCI) Cancer Information Service (1-800-4-CANCER) can give you the names of NCI-affiliated clinical or comprehensive cancer centers in your state. Call and ask them for a referral or, if they are conveniently located, consider consulting a physician on their staff.
- Divisions and units of the American Cancer Society will often provide local referrals. You may also call the national office of the society at 1-800-ACS-2345 for such information.
- The American College of Surgeons (312-664-4050) will give you names of surgeons specializing in breast cancer in your area.
- Find out if there is a local women's health group or women's center. Such groups often know of doctors in the area who specialize in women's health problems. They sometimes keep records of women's experiences—good and bad—with local doctors.
- Call the best hospital in your region and ask for the names of breast cancer specialists. If there are several such people on staff, you may simply be given the names of the people next in order on the hospital's list. Still, this may be a useful place to start your search.
- Call your clergyman or a social worker at a mental health ser-

vice. Such people may know the names of good physicians in the community or may know other cancer patients who have had the experience of looking for and finding a doctor.

How Do You Evaluate the Physicians Whose Names You Now Have?

One way to get started "checking out" a doctor is to consult the medical directories that are available at public libraries, at the county medical society offices, or at medical libraries. State medical societies usually publish annual or biannual listings that describe a physician's training, specialty, and current hospital affiliation. There is also a directory of medical specialists that will give you such information.

The first factor to consider is *training.* This is one of the simplest pieces of your detective work. If you are in the doctor's office, she may have her diplomas and degrees on the wall. Take note of what institutions they are from. If you don't see these documents, ask the doctor where she trained, or else consult one of the directories or listings described above. The medical school a physician attended is often less important than where she took her postgraduate or specialty training. The best training usually is at large, university-affiliated hospitals (often called teaching hospitals). Institutions like these treat many patients and they also maintain high standards. There is usually additional training available specifically in cancer surgery and other cancer treatment.

The next factor to concern yourself with is *experience.* This is not to say that a smart young doctor, fresh out of training at a great institution, very sharp about the latest techniques, can't do a good job. There is, however, for better or worse, a demonstrable correlation between, for example, the outcome of the surgery and the surgeon's experience in doing the procedure. The frequency of postoperative complications often is related to how many times the surgeon has performed a particular operation.

Hospital affiliation is another crucial issue. Make sure that the physician is on the staff of a hospital known to have both very high standards and good support services for the treatment of

25

breast cancer patients. This is important not only because you want to be treated at the best possible institution, but also because the fact that a physician practices at such a hospital shows that the best doctors in the community acknowledge his qualifications by accepting him as a colleague.

If you live in a very small community—without a hospital of this caliber and a pool of cancer specialists from whom to choose—you should seriously consider seeking diagnosis and treatment in a large regional hospital or in a nearby large city. Even if that won't be possible for the entire course of your treatment, it's what you should try for at the time of the diagnosis, surgery, and the planning of the treatment.

There are hospitals and medical centers that are specifically devoted to the treatment of cancer. The Dana Farber Cancer Center in Boston, Memorial Sloan-Kettering Cancer Center in New York, and the M. D. Anderson Cancer Center in Houston are among these.

Some women so badly want to be treated at a hospital that is a cancer center that—if they don't already know an affiliated physician—they accept as their doctor anyone to whom the institution assigns them. There's little doubt that they'll get competent care, but that method of picking a doctor doesn't feel right to me. The most important consideration is to find a physician who is experienced, whose reputation among patients as well as other doctors is exemplary, whose approach to your case is carefully and thoughtfully arrived at, and who has your interests at heart.

Peer recognition—what his colleagues think of a doctor's abilities—is harder to find out, but a very useful piece of information. Doctors, as all nondoctors recognize, are reluctant to say directly unfavorable things about their colleagues. You may need to make such inquiries more subtly. For example, ask several doctors in the community who they think is the best breast surgeon in town. The same names will probably recur. If the physician you're investigating isn't mentioned, you already know a lot, but you might want to push this a little further by asking, "Do you think Dr. Jackson is in the same league?" You may have to watch closely here for the slight shake of the head, or put your ear tightly to the phone receiver to hear the meaningful pause or clearing of the throat. Though there aren't too many doctors who will be immediately forthcoming, responsible physicians will try to protect you from people, particularly surgeons, whose work is not first-rate.

As alluded to before, the opinion of *other women who have had breast cancer* is invaluable. This includes former patients of the physicians you are considering. Many of my patients point out that they often get phone calls from women who have heard through the grapevine that they had cancer. These people call and ask, "Whom did you go to?" "What kind of operation did you have?" and similar questions. A former patient's opinion should probably not be the only basis for making a decision to go to a particular doctor. If, however, a few women tell you of unpleasant or bad experiences with a doctor, that is a good reason *not* to go to him, or, at the very least, to do a lot more investigation.

Approach to the Disease

One of the hardest questions to judge when you have breast cancer is whether the treatment that is being proposed is the right one for you. This is especially difficult because individual women may have specific goals of their own and may not know how to reconcile them with what they are being told is the proper course to follow.

A woman may say, "The most important thing for me is to preserve my breast." Another, perhaps expressing her hope for a normal, unimpaired life, will say, "I want to be able to go on playing tennis." Another will say, "The only thing that matters to me is survival. Cut off my breast tomorrow if that means I'll be safe."

These are important concerns, though obviously the primary factor that should determine treatment is the extent and nature of the illness. Given a particular patient's situation, however, there may be differences of opinion among physicians on what the treatment should be. A good doctor should be able to explain to you the principle on which he wishes to proceed and the interpretation that has led him to propose a course of action.

Why, given a certain condition, wouldn't every physician you see suggest the same treatment plan? Some women report running into doctors who seem to have a bias toward one treatment or the other; who, despite recent research and clinical experience, are slow to change; or who are especially cautious. Women have told me that such doctors have said, for example, "I never do lumpectomies. They're risky."

Nonetheless, there are genuine differences in how to "call" a case. Suppose removing the entire breast in one circumstance would result in a one hundred percent chance of success, while doing a wide excision (lumpectomy) followed by radiation would yield a ninety-seven percent success rate. In such a case, the advice of two different physicians might legitimately differ.

If an opinion does not seem reasonable to you or if you are particularly anxious about a recommended course of treatment, consult another doctor (as your insurance company may require you to). The second physician may confirm that what is being planned is the only sound course of action; or you may have to choose between two conflicting opinions, or even seek a third specialist's advice. Even though this sounds troublesome, you owe it to yourself to be as sure as possible before you undergo an extensive procedure.

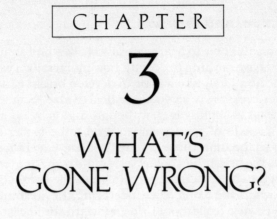

3

WHAT'S
GONE WRONG?

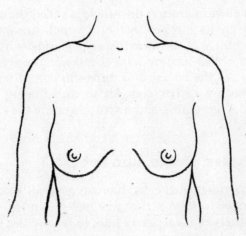

WHAT IS THE BREAST?

The breast is a gland, the mammary gland, designed by nature to
produce milk so that a woman can feed her infant.

Size, Shape, and Position

Though breasts come in a large variety of sizes and shapes, these differences have nothing to do with how much milk a woman can produce or how likely she will be to develop breast cancer.

The two breasts are seldom identical in size. In many women the left breast is slightly larger, though that is by no means the rule. The breasts of young women tend to be firmer and more conical in shape than those of older women. Except for those in the nipple, the breast has no muscles of its own, but rests on the muscles of the chest wall, the pectoral muscles. Breast tissue also extends toward the axilla (the underarm), the sternum (breast-bone), the clavicle (collarbone), down toward the lowest ribs, and back toward the latissimus dorsi (the muscle at the side).

Nipple

The nipple is slightly below the centerpoint of the breast. Darker than the rest of the breast, its color varies from woman to woman. It becomes erect when it is stimulated, providing a firm protuberance for the baby to suck on. The nipple also becomes erect and may increase in size during lovemaking. Like the entire breast, the nipple changes considerably during pregnancy and lactation, becoming larger and darker in color.

Areola

The pigmented skin around the nipple is called the areola. It has tiny bumps on its surface, some of which are sweat glands, others the endings of the Montgomery's glands, which lubricate the nipple for breast-feeding. Like the nipple, the areola is darker than the rest of the breast and differs in color from woman to woman according to her complexion and during the various stages of life. A darkening of the areola is one of the earliest signs of pregnancy.

Acini, Lobules, Ducts, and Lobes

Acini are sacs lined with cells that can produce milk. The acini cluster together to form structures called lobules. The lobules empty into ducts that can carry milk to the nipple. The group of

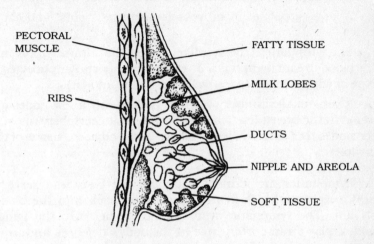

PECTORAL
MUSCLE

FATTY TISSUE

MILK LOBES

RIBS

DUCTS

NIPPLE AND AREOLA

SOFT TISSUE

Cross section of the breast

lobules that empty into any one duct is called a lobe. This milk-producing system is, of course, not normally activated until childbirth.

It is useful to think of this system as a tree: the major ducts that end in the nipple constitute the trunk; as the ducts become finer, they resemble branches that spread throughout the breast, back from the nipple, and end in the lobules, which are like the leaves of the tree.

Fat

The breast is cushioned with fat that protects its important milk-producing organs. In fact, the breast is mainly composed of fat. In very small breasts there is so little fat that on examination you feel mainly glandular tissue, but the breast's composition is seldom less than one-third fat. As a woman ages, glandular tissue, no longer needed for infant-feeding, is replaced by fat.

Other Breast Components

The breast is also composed of these elements:

Connective tissue called fascia that enclose and support it

A large supply of blood vessels—arteries, veins, and capillaries

The lymphatics, the veinlike vessels that drain lymph into the bloodstream (lymph is a fluid that transports lymphocytes, a type of white blood cell, as well as proteins and fat)

A very small number of lymph nodes (only a few nodes are found in the breast itself, and these are on its periphery; most of the nodes that service the breast are in the adjacent tissue of the armpit)

Lymphatics are found throughout the body and serve to drain extracellular fluid from the tissue back into the bloodstream. The lymphatic system, and particularly the lymph nodes, play an important role in the body's defenses and in its immune system. In the area of the breast, the lymphatics go from the breast and nipple to the nodes in the armpit and from there to the nodes above the collarbone. The central and inner part of the breast, however, can also drain to nodes under the breastbone.

WHAT IS BREAST CANCER?

Assume, as a way to get started, that you have been told that you have breast cancer or that it is suspected, or that it must be ruled out. What does this mean? What *is* cancer?

Cancer

Cancer is not just one disease. It can appear in any part of the body and can take many forms. All of them involve the abnormal multiplication and spread of cells in the body. This unrestrained growth is caused by a genetic change in the cells that also empowers them to move from their normal locale to other parts of the body.

The abnormal growth of cells often results in the formation of a tumor. Benign tumors, which are discussed on pages 40–45, can result from a limited loss of growth control of the cells. But when the growth is rampantly out of control, and when the cells have the ability to move from their original site and settle and grow in other tissues, the condition is cancer, a malignancy.

The term used for the most common types of cancer, and for most malignant tumors, is **carcinoma.** A **sarcoma** is the term used to describe a tumor originating in bone, muscle, fat, or connective tissue.

Carcinoma of the breast occurs when this malignant change takes place in the cells that line the lobules that manufacture milk or, more commonly, in the ducts that carry it to the nipple. Since most of these cells are found in the upper part of the breast, in the outer quadrant, or in the area around the center of the breast, these are the locations in which most cancers occur. It is rare for tumors to originate in the fat or nonglandular tissues of the breast. When they do, they are called sarcomas.

PHYSICAL CHARACTERISTICS

Any tumor is first examined physically in order to decide whether it is "likely" to be cancer. What is its shape? Terms such as *well-delineated, irregular,* or *diffuse* are used to describe the contours of the tumor. Is it *hard* or *soft*? *Movable* or *fixed*?

In general, a tumor is more likely to be malignant if it is firm and irregular in shape. Those factors do not always mean that cancer is present, but they do make us suspect this, and they lead us to the final step in our investigation, an examination of the cells under a microscope by a pathologist (see Chapter Five). These cells are obtained from a biopsy, which is discussed on pages 69–80.

From the pathological examination, the cancer is classified by such characteristics as the pattern in which it grows, the arrangement of the cells, their variety in size and shape, the frequency with which they divide, and also by the presence on their surface of receptors for the hormones estrogen and progesterone. (See Chapter Five.)

Kinds of Breast Cancer

As noted, most cancers in the breast originate in the ducts, and are called ductal or duct cell carcinoma. A much smaller number originate in the lobules: lobular carcinoma. When we look at the cancer cells through a microscope, we usually can identify them as either ductal or lobular, although sometimes both types may be present.

A few ductal or lobular tumors have a specific appearance or pattern that can be identified under a microscope. These tumors have been named and grouped into subcategories that include *tubular, medullary, mucinous, papillary,* and *adenocystic.* You may hear these terms in the doctor's office, but the percentage of women who have any particular one of these cancers is relatively small. It should also be said that the prognosis for women with these cancers is excellent.

IN SITU CANCERS

If the cancer cells remain within the confines of the duct or lobule, within what you may hear referred to as the basement membrane, it is called an **in situ cancer,** meaning it is confined "in that site." These cancers have not formed a tumor mass and therefore cannot be felt during a physical examination. They are detected by mammography. (See page 57.)

In situ cancers are sometimes referred to as precancerous. This is not an accurate term and I consider its use dangerous. *In situ* cancer cells multiply like other malignancies, though they may be slower-growing. They are not life-threatening if they are treated promptly, but *they are cancer.* They must get prompt attention—or the advantage of early detection will be lost and a more serious illness may result.

In situ cancers of the duct were rarely seen until mammography screening became more common in recent years and mammography techniques so refined. The result is that we are able to find tiny, very early cancers of this type and to treat them very successfully.

In situ cancers of the lobules are often discovered incidentally during a biopsy when we are investigating a minimal thickening or subtle abnormality. This type of *in situ* cancer is most common in premenopausal women, and there is some likelihood that if this cancer appears in one breast, it may also occur in the other. For that reason, if a lobular carcinoma *in situ* is found, the second breast should be watched particularly carefully.

INFILTRATING CANCERS

If the cancer cells have penetrated the membrane that surrounds the duct or lobule, they are said to be **infiltrating,** or **invasive,** and they eventually form a lump that can be felt on physical examination. Very early infiltrating cancers, however, may be detected only on a mammogram.

INFILTRATING CANCER OF THE DUCT

This cancer, which you may hear referred to as infiltrating ductal carcinoma, is the most common type of breast cancer and is the cause of many of the signs we normally associate with breast cancer.

As the cancer cells invade the fatty tissue around the duct, they stimulate the growth of fibrous, noncancerous, scarlike tissue that surrounds the cancer. Thus, the actual size of the cancer is often smaller than the size of the lump may suggest. A welcome result of this thickening is that it makes the mass easier to find during physical examination as well as on a mammogram.

Depending on the location of the ductal cancer, it may cause the nipple to retract, or it may result in a nipple discharge, or skin changes such as puckering or dimpling. These symptoms may also be caused by other benign conditions (see below), but they are a signal that warrants prompt investigation.

INFILTRATING CANCER OF THE LOBULES

This condition, also called infiltrating lobular carcinoma, occurs when cells stream out in single file into the surrounding breast tissue. About fifteen percent of breast cancers originate in the lobules.

Because it does not provoke the kind of fibrous growth we see in ductal cancer, and so may be harder to detect on a mammogram, cancer of the lobule is likely to be larger than ductal cancer when it is first detected. It also feels softer and is likely to be described as a thickening rather than as a lump.

As we have discussed, if we find a lobular cancer in one breast, it may be present in the other breast as well. For this reason, the second breast should be watched and a biopsy performed if a mammogram reveals any suspicious findings or if a lump develops. You should discuss this with your surgeon if a lobular cancer is found.

PAGET'S DISEASE

A tumor close to the nipple will sometimes be detected because of scaliness, oozing, or hardening of the skin of the areola or the nipple itself, or because of an ulcer on the nipple's surface. Though the problem may prove to be a simple eczema that responds to local treatment, a biopsy must be performed to rule out the presence of the malignant cells that are characteristic of this relatively rare cancer. If these Paget cells are found, it usually indicates that there is an underlying *in situ* or invasive ductal cancer in the breast.

CYSTOSARCOMA PHYLLODES

This rare malignant breast tumor usually appears in women in their thirties and forties, often after a history of rapidly recurring fibroadenomas, benign lumps discussed on page 44. The tumor seems very like a fibroadenoma when it is excised, but when it is examined under a microscope, we see many elongated cells that originate in the fibrous tissue of the breast and resemble a sarcoma.

Though they do not usually spread to other parts of the body, the edges of a cystosarcoma tend to invade the adjacent breast tissue, and these tumors also tend to recur locally. For these reasons, when we remove the tumor, we also remove a rim of normal tissue around it. If a cystosarcoma is large or if it recurs, a mastectomy may be necessary.

INFLAMMATORY CANCER

This uncommon condition accounts for only about one percent of all breast cancers and usually presents itself as a swollen and reddened breast that may look as if there is an infection present. There is usually no lump and the condition does not respond to antibiotics. When a biopsy is performed, cancer cells are found. The breast is inflamed because this aggressive cancer has spread to the lymphatics in the skin, where it induces a pink discoloration.

BREAST CANCER DURING PREGNANCY

Unfortunately, we are now seeing more breast cancer in pregnant women than we did in the past. That is probably because the rate of breast cancer has been increasing for all women in recent years, and also because many women are delaying their pregnancies until ages when breast cancer begins to become more common.

Pregnancy is usually a happy time in a woman's life. She's not thinking about breast cancer; she's also not examining her breasts to look for it. Nor, probably, is her doctor. Moreover, her breasts are swelling and changing in contour in the normal course of the pregnancy. For that reason, breast cancer tends to be found at a relatively later stage in pregnant women.

We used to think that pregnant women did more poorly than other women with breast cancer because of the increased hormonal activity of pregnancy. Now we have learned that if compared stage by stage, the results are about the same for pregnant women as for others with breast cancer. The problem, as we have noted, is that in pregnant women treatment is initiated at a later stage of the disease. (For a discussion of the treatment of breast cancer during pregnancy, see page 129.)

SIZE AND SPREAD

Among the most crucial considerations of a cancerous tumor have to do with how big it is and how much it has spread. Here, the common-sense conclusion is the right one: we hope for a small tumor, under two centimeters in size (about three-quarters of an inch), which has not spread to the lymph nodes or to a distant site (has not metastasized).

Having said that, it is important to note that it isn't until a tumor is over five centimeters (about two inches) or more in size that it gets to be called large, and also that some women with long-standing large lesions do well.

The spread of breast cancer is usually referred to in the following ways:

- *Local*, meaning it is confined within the breast, though it may be in several locations there
- *Regional*, meaning that the lymph nodes, primarily those in the armpit, are involved

37

- *Distant*, meaning the cancer is found in other parts of the body as well

The Classification of Cancer

Why do these classifications and fine distinctions matter? Why, if you have cancer, don't we just get on with the treatment? To a woman facing breast cancer, this certainly feels like the first priority.

Patience is important here, for both the woman and her physician. This is true even though diagnosis may take longer than we would like. The reason as precise an identification as possible is important—of the cell type, its differentiation, tumor size, the relationship to adjacent breast tissue, and the spread to adjacent or distant places in the body—is because these are the factors that affect risk and that make it possible to determine what ought to be done to treat the patient most effectively.

The system of classifying cancer is complicated, and there are variations in the methods and criteria from country to country, region to region, and sometimes even from medical center to medical center. The explanations that follow, drawn from an international classification system, have been limited to what you may hear in the doctor's office, or read about, as well as what you need to know in order to join your physician in assessing your risk and in choosing the treatment that is appropriate for you.

TUMORS

Tumors are classified primarily by certain standard characteristics:

A. Have the cancer cells demonstrated the ability to leave their site of origin? *In situ* cancer cells, which have multiplied within a duct or lobule but remain confined to that site, are less likely to metastasize than cells that have begun to infiltrate normal breast tissue.

B. How big is the tumor? When the cells invade the breast fat and form a tumor, we consider the size.

C. What is the condition of the skin over the tumor site? Is it broken? retracted? swollen?

D. Has the nipple retracted into the breast or does it still protrude?

E. Is the tumor attached to the pectoral muscle or the chest wall?

You also may hear of the designations T*is*, T1, T2, T3, or T4 in connection with tumors. These simply mean the tumor is being rated according to the criteria described above. The simplified list that follows will help us begin to examine this rating system:

Tis is an *in situ* tumor.

T1 is a small tumor, under two centimeters in size.

T2 is a tumor two to five centimeters.

T3 is a tumor over five centimeters.

T4 is a tumor of *any* size that is accompanied by any of the following characteristics: tumor fixed to the pectoral muscle or to the chest wall; involvement of the lymphatics within the *skin* of the breast (not within the breast itself); infiltration of the skin by malignant cells; skin ulceration. (Note that the tumor may be situated in such a way that it pulls the skin or causes the nipple to retract. It is not a T4 tumor unless the skin itself is invaded.)

LYMPH NODES

After biopsy, the lymph nodes in the armpit (axilla) are classified:

N0 means there is no cancer present.

N1 means there is cancer involvement but the nodes are movable, not fixed in place by the spread of cancer.

N2 means the nodes are attached to one another or to adjacent blood vessels.

N3 means there is spread to the nodes above the collarbone.

METASTASIS

Metastasis, or spreading, must be evaluated next. Has the cancer spread from the breast to the underarm lymph nodes? Is it now present elsewhere in the body? The cancer is said to have metastasized if it has spread beyond the area of the breast and the axillary lymph nodes into other parts of the body.

THE STAGES

The conditions we've been describing—of the *T*umor, the lymph *N*odes, and *M*etastasis—are taken into account in order to determine the stage at which the cancer has been found. This is called the **TNM system** of staging. Staging is a vital tool in measuring risk and in choosing treatment.

When the tumor is small, the lymph nodes are not involved, and there is no metastasis, the cancer is considered Stage I. The other end of the scale, Stage IV, describes the situation where the cancer has spread to a site far from the original tumor. Stage II and Stage III fall between those two ends.

Classifying into these stages means evaluating all factors related to TNM. A woman might have a quite small tumor, but also involvement of the lymph nodes. Conversely, the tumor may be large but confined to one area, with no evidence of spread. The various combinations of these factors are considered together to determine the extent and stage of the disease.

The following chart very neatly sets out the combinations of characteristics of the tumor (T); the nodes (N); and the metastasis (M) that make up the stages. N0, for example, means there is no node involvement. M1 means that there is metastasis to a distant site. Note that Stages II and III on this chart have been further broken down into IIA and IIB.

This material is the stuff of the cancer specialist: when the stage of the cancer is precisely determined, we can assess the risk and choose the appropriate treatment.

You should know the terminology not only because you may hear or read about it, but because it will help you understand and evaluate the reasons for the treatment that is being suggested for you.

IT MAY NOT BE CANCER AFTER ALL

Not every breast problem is cancer, nor is every lump. In fact, about ninety percent of lumps or other suspicious breast changes turn out to be benign tumors or cysts. You should carefully investigate each abnormality, as we will see in Chapter

Stage Groupings*

	Classification		
Stage	T	N	M
0	Tis	N0	M0
I	T1	N0	M0
IIA	T0	N1	M0
	T1	N1	M0
	T2	N0	M0
IIB	T2	N1	M0
	T3	N0	M0
IIIA	T0	N2	M0
	T1	N2	M0
	T2	N2	M0
	T3	N1, N2	M0
IIIB	T4	Any N	M0
	Any T	N3	M0
IV	Any T	Any N	M1

Four on diagnosis, but in most instances, these conditions will prove not to be serious enough to be a source of worry.

Cancer is only one of several causes of lumps or other irregularities of breast shape. The other common conditions that may account for such problems follow.

---

* Adapted from the American Joint Committee on Cancer: *Manual for Staging of Cancer.* Fourth Edition, 1992. Philadelphia: J. B. Lippincott Company. Reprinted by permission.

BREAST CYSTS OR GROSS CYSTIC DISEASE

A cyst is a sac filled with fluid. You or someone you know has probably had a cyst sometime during your life, perhaps on the eyelid or the gum. Such cysts are lined with cells that produce secretions. They are usually surgically removed.

Breast cysts are different. They are really dilated, pinched-off sections of ducts that "passively" fill up with fluid, rather than manufacturing it themselves. They do not ordinarily have to be surgically removed.

Breast cysts are usually first observed in women in their late twenties and thirties. They rarely develop in women past menopause. The chances are that if you develop one cyst, you're likely to develop more. Women prone to cysts will find that the cysts tend to shrink or disappear after menopause.

Typically round and evenly contoured, breast cysts may also be movable. They may change quite dramatically in size during the menstrual cycle. They can be extremely small or quite large, as much as five centimeters or more in diameter.

Though some women experience pain or tenderness with breast cysts, particularly around the time they menstruate, most often there are no accompanying symptoms. You usually find out you have a cyst because you or your doctor discovers a lump in your breast. A lump must be investigated. It shouldn't be there.

The doctor will aspirate the lump by injecting a small amount of anesthetic into the skin, inserting a hollow needle, and drawing out the fluid. The mass should disappear. If it does, it was a cyst. If it doesn't, or if fluid cannot be withdrawn, the lump should be surgically removed and examined. That does *not* mean that it is cancer. It may only mean that it is a cyst that, for reason of its position or other factors, could not be successfully aspirated.

Any fluid that is aspirated from the cyst is examined by the doctor. If it is tan or greenish in color, which is considered typical of cyst fluid, there is nothing more to be learned from it and the doctor can simply throw it away.

If, however, the fluid is golden-colored or tinged with blood, it should be examined by a pathologist because it may indicate the presence of a rare cystic cancer.

If cysts, after they are aspirated, tend to recur in the same place over a period of years, they should probably be surgically removed. There is some evidence that women with recurrent cysts are at a slightly higher risk of developing breast cancer after menopause.

There remains a fair amount of controversy about whether the repeated appearance of large cysts places a woman at higher risk for getting cancer. At this moment, no one knows for sure. We do know, however, that the converse isn't true: many women who do get breast cancer have never had such cysts.

In my opinion the question should be put slightly differently. There is the very practical problem that in women who have fairly lumpy breasts, it may be hard to distinguish *new* lumps or, in fact, to distinguish between cysts and cancerous tumors. And a cyst, by its position or size, may "hide" a malignancy.

FIBROCYSTIC DISEASE (FORMERLY CALLED CYSTIC MASTITIS)

Sometimes used when a woman is prone to small cysts, the terms *fibrocystic disease* and *cystic mastitis* would best be put to rest. They are "nondiseases." In the monthly changes in the breasts as they prepare for pregnancy and then "turn off," ducts may pinch off, inflammations may come and go. Very rarely do these changes result in the risk of cancer.

Physicians often tell women they are "cystic" because they have painful or lumpy breasts. Having a lot of cysts or "lumpiness" in the breast can be uncomfortable and cause concern. The lumps may swell and become tender before menstruation and then shrink or even seem to disappear once the period begins. But these are not indications of malignancy or of life-threatening disease.

There is, however, one caution to be mentioned here: sometimes a lumpy area is surgically removed and the pathologist's conclusion from his postsurgery examination (see page 82) is "fibrocystic disease." He may tell us that he has seen under a microscope a condition called **hyperplasia** (meaning there are too many cells in the tissue he's examining) or **atypia** (meaning that the appearance of the cells is unusual, "atypical"). In only a very small percentage of these cases does this indicate an important abnormality or a risk of the future development of cancer. In

43

both instances, however, the condition should be closely monitored.

FIBROADENOMAS

The term *fibroadenoma* is used to describe an orderly growth of cells, confined to the breast, that results in benign, movable, and rounded lumps. Rounded lumps in teenagers and young women are almost always fibroadenomas. Because these lumps tend to grow, they are usually removed. Since the risk of breast cancer increases with age, any such breast masses definitely should be removed and examined through biopsy in women over twenty.

INFECTIONS

Various infections, several of them associated with pregnancy and nursing, occur in the breast and can be successfully treated with antibiotics. These disorders include bacterial mastitis and abscesses.

A more persistent problem called chronic subareolar infection is found just around the areola, in the central part of the breast. It tends to be recurrent, and treatment with antibiotics should begin as soon as possible. As with any abscess, the site may need to be surgically opened and drained.

FAT NECROSIS

When, for a variety of reasons, the cells of an area of the breast die, a small, hard, flat lump may appear. This condition, called fat necrosis, is usually seen in women over fifty and is benign; but because we also see an increase in breast cancer in women of this age, a biopsy should be performed. Obviously, a diagnosis of fat necrosis, or "destruction" of some fat cells, comes as a great relief. The condition does not cause any problems and requires no further treatment.

INTRADUCTAL PAPILLOMA

Intraductal papillomas are tiny, polyplike, benign growths that occur, frequently several at a time, in the ducts behind the nipple. Intraductal papilloma is the usual cause of a watery or bloody discharge from the nipple. Because such a discharge may also be a warning sign of cancer, it should be investigated by biopsy as soon as possible. To do that, the affected ducts are removed, commonly during an outpatient procedure in the hospital.

MAMMARY DUCT ECTASIA

Mammary duct ectasia is a benign condition in the ductal system in which the ducts become distended and clogged. Usually occurring in women in their forties, the problem may present itself as a lump, there may be swelling and a nipple discharge, and an area of the breast may become inflamed. Because this disorder can look so much like cancer, you must make sure that a biopsy is performed so that on the one hand, it is confirmed that you do not have cancer; and on the other hand, you are not treated as if you do, with more heroic measures than are necessary. Sometimes the inflammation caused by this disorder will go away on its own. If it is troublesome, or if the symptoms keep recurring, you and your doctor may want to discuss the advisability of localized surgery to correct the problem.

MONDOR'S DISEASE

An inflamed vein or phlebitis of the breast can cause a fairly superficial lump and a drawing sensation that sometimes radiates down toward the abdomen. This condition, called Mondor's disease, is self-limiting, and is treated with heat.

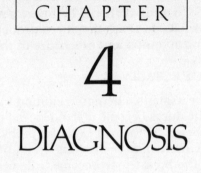

CHAPTER

4

DIAGNOSIS

We've now considered the normal breast and the various things that can go wrong with it. How do you use that information to ascertain what is going on in your own body when you suspect there may be a problem or when, in fact, a lump has been found?

Breast lumps are usually discovered in one of three ways: women find them themselves; they are discovered by a doctor during a physical examination; or they are detected on a mammogram, a special X-ray examination of the breast. If all women were having routine mammography, 85 percent of all breast cancers would be found by X ray (see page 57).

If you have found a lump yourself, you're in good company. It may seem startling, but most malignant lumps are still found by women themselves, either through self-examination or else by chance. This observation is a humbling one for doctors.

Why are women such experts? Because they know how their own bodies normally feel at various times during the month. They know the contours of their own breasts, and they are therefore in the best position to notice any changes. It naturally follows that the more familiar you are with your breasts, the better prepared you are to detect any changes.

The first step in identifying potential problems is to learn as much about your own breasts as you can. Breast self-examination (sometimes referred to as BSE) is the best way to do that, though being alert to your breast contours even when you're not specifically examining them can be extremely useful. Many women have found a suspicious lump when they were washing themselves in the shower or scratching a mosquito bite. Even "accidental" discoveries such as these, however, are much more likely if you have already learned the topography of your breast through self-examination.

Sometimes, either accidentally or in deliberately examining your breasts, you may notice that there is a painful spot. This is not at all uncommon. There is an old saying, "If it hurts, it's not cancer." That's usually true, but in a very small percentage of cases, cancerous lumps do hurt. You should call the painful place to your physician's attention.

BREAST SELF-EXAMINATION

A reminder of a fact already stated is useful here: about ninety percent of all breast lumps turn out to be benign. By learning the techniques of self-examination, you are not specifically learning how to discover a cancer. You are learning to spot changes in your breasts that may or may not mean trouble—mostly "not."

Another comforting fact: describing this monthly procedure may make it sound more complicated and time-consuming than it actually is. After all, most people in our society have a daily routine which, if it were outlined in detail, would sound as if we had no time during the day to do more than our morning and evening toilet. Think of all the separate steps in flossing and brushing our teeth, taking a bath, combing our hair, keeping our fingernails trimmed, taking vitamins, shaving, putting our contact lenses in and taking them out, et cetera.

This list sounds ludicrous, because we've done all these things so often that they are built into our daily schedule. We don't have to mark on our calendar, "7:30, brush teeth." The aim now should be to make breast self-examination as much a part of your life routine as brushing your teeth—except that you only have to do it once a month, not twice a day.

When it is done properly, breast self-examination can significantly reduce the risk of advanced-stage cancer. Unfortunately, most women do not know the proper technique. Learning it could greatly increase the possibility of detecting a cancer in its early stages.

A Time Schedule for Breast Self-Examination

AT WHAT AGE SHOULD I BEGIN?

A good time to start is in the late teens or early twenties. That's usually when women first visit a gynecologist or a women's health facility, and this is a convenient opportunity to begin to learn how to perform self-examination and to incorporate the habit into your life.

WHEN CAN I STOP SELF-EXAMINATION?

Never. It is, as we'll see, an easy thing to do, and you should continue the procedure throughout your life, especially since breast cancer becomes more common as you get older.

HOW OFTEN SHOULD I EXAMINE MY BREASTS?

You must examine your breasts, carefully and thoroughly, once a month. In addition to this scheduled, thorough examination, however, you'll find that as you become familiar with the appearance and contours of your breasts, you'll also be a more alert observer of any changes that may take place between examinations.

48

WHEN DURING THE MONTH SHOULD
I DO MY EXAM?

We tie the timing of self-examination to the menstrual cycle because the breast's texture and contour often change during the month. You may have noticed that a few days before you get your period, the breasts become firmer and fuller. They also can become tender—in some women slightly so, in others quite painfully. The breasts may feel lumpy at that time of the month—"nodular," your doctor may call it. This is a natural result of premenstrual engorgement. It does not indicate a cyst or a cancerous lump. The swelling, tenderness, and lumpiness will almost certainly disappear after you menstruate. For these reasons, you should not perform your regular breast self-examination just before your menstrual period.

Examine your breasts every month, ten days after the start of your period. If you miss the tenth day, do your examination as soon afterward as you can. Do not wait until the next month to "catch up."

Postmenopausal women should examine their breasts on the first day of every month.

Some women who are not yet of menopause age have had a hysterectomy, with their uterus removed but one or both ovaries retained. If you are in that situation, you may feel your body going through the various stages of the menstrual cycle even though you don't actually menstruate. Choose a regular time each month when your breasts are not swollen for your self-examination.

THE ELEMENTS OF BREAST
SELF-EXAMINATION

There are two general aspects of examining your breasts: what you see and what you feel.

Visual Observation

Remember: you are not looking for cancer. You are studying your breasts, first, to observe their *normal* appearance so that you will have a reference point in the future from which you can spot something new. You are also looking for changes from what you may only casually have observed in the past or for conditions that seem to you unusual for your normal breast.

What is "normal" differs from person to person. As we have noted, in many women the breasts are of slightly different size. The nipple may be in a different place on each breast. One or both nipples may be somewhat retracted—that is, pulled inside. In order to identify changes, you would need to have noted such normal details of the appearance of your breasts.

THE STEPS

1. Take off your blouse and bra and stand about two feet in front of a mirror that has a good, clear image.

2. Put your hands at your sides and observe the general contour of each breast.
   - Is the shape of the breast even, without any visible swelling or distortion?
   - Are both breasts their usual size?
   - Is the nipple in the same position on each breast?
   - Do the nipples protrude or is one or both of them retracted?
   - Do your breasts appear different in any way from the last time you looked at them?

3. Now raise your arms above your head.
   - Do you see any dimpling of the skin?
   - Is there a rash of any type?
   - Are there other changes in the skin's surface?

4. Place your hands on your hips and, flexing your shoulders forward, continue to visually observe the surface of the skin as described above.

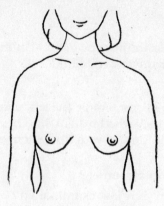 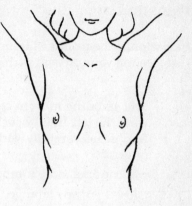

[1] *Observe your breasts in a mirror.*

[2] *Raise your arms above your head.*

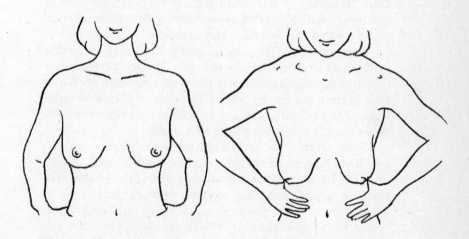

[3] *Place your hands on your hips.*

[4] *Flex your shoulders forward.*

Breast self-examination

Palpation

Palpation is the technical term for examining by touch—in this case, feeling your breasts with your fingers and hand.

1. Still standing in front of the mirror, cradle the left breast with the left hand beneath it. With the right hand, feel the breast carefully with the tips of your three longest fingers.
   - Is one area more lumpy than any other?
   - Are there any changes from your last examination?

2. Now cradle the right breast and repeat this palpation.

3. Lie down, flat on your back, with a pillow under your right shoulder. Stretch your right arm behind you, bend your elbow, and put your hand behind your head.

   Again using the pads of the three longest fingers of your left hand, examine your right breast from the edge of the nipple out to the rim of your breast and then up your chest toward the shoulder and armpit.

   Keep pressing the tissue, going clockwise in circles that spiral from the areola out. Use enough pressure on the skin so that you can feel the tissue beneath it. While your fingers are on the breast, move them back and forth slightly to seek out irregularities. If you are full-breasted, be especially careful to probe thoroughly.

   Some women prefer to examine their breasts by moving their fingers in overlapping vertical "strips," going from the breastbone to the side, covering the breast and the area approaching the shoulder and armpit.

   Others conduct their examination by thinking of the breast as being divided into wedges, like a pie. They examine each wedge from the nipple out, and then back again.

   Any one of these methods is acceptable as long as you carefully cover the entire area of the breast and of the chest as it approaches the shoulder and the armpit.

4. Now repeat the palpation of the left breast.

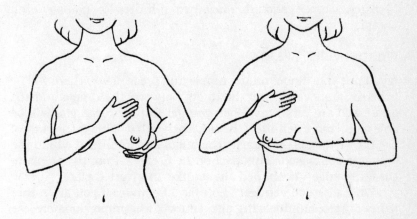

[1] *Cradle the left breast and gently feel it with the fingers of your right hand.*

[2] *Cradle the right breast and repeat this palpation.*

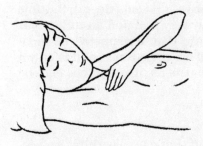

[3] *Lying down with your right hand behind your head, palpate the right breast with the fingers of your left hand.*

[4] *Repeat this procedure with the left breast.*

After the first couple of times you do this examination, it will take less time, but do not rush through the process. Even small-breasted women should allow two minutes to palpate each breast.

WHAT SHOULD I FEEL?

If you put your finger on the nipple and press down, there will be little resistance because the ducts between the nipple and the chest wall are very fine. When you get to the areola, you will be able to feel more definitely the ridge beneath it. This is the start of the firmer tissue—primarily the ducts and lobules of which the breast is composed. This part of the breast—from the areola to the outer edge—is shaped almost like an inverted plate.

What else will you feel? Soft fat, of course. If you are rather thin or are of childbearing age, you will feel proportionately less fat and more breast tissue.

Some women will feel a lump or the kind of nodularity described earlier. *This should be checked by a physician the first time you feel it.* However, after you have had a professional examination of your lump or "lumpiness" and have been told the condition is not a cause for concern, you will learn to differentiate between irregularities that are simply part of your own physiology and those that are new.

As we have seen, if you examine your breasts close to the time of your menstrual period, you may very well find an unfamiliar thickening. The changes in texture that accompany the menstrual cycle are to be expected and are of no concern. It is only a fresh lump, which persists during the month, that needs to be investigated.

NIPPLE DISCHARGE

Though some physicians suggest it, I don't really think it's necessary during your regular self-examination to squeeze your nipple to look for a discharge.

If, however, you observe a discharge in the course of your examination, or if a discharge is apparent at other times during the month, *then* squeeze the nipple. Do this a few times over the course of several days. If the discharge continues, consult a doctor.

THE ARMPIT

If you have a cold or other infection, the glands under your arm may be slightly tender. You may have a blocked sweat gland under your arm that becomes irritated. Sometimes there is breast tissue in the armpit, and it may swell during the menstrual cycle or during pregnancy like other breast tissue. Very rarely, an enlarged lymph node is the first sign of breast cancer. If you notice a lump in this area, have a physician look at it just to be sure that nothing is amiss.

Training in Breast Self-Examination

It would be ideal to have a doctor go through the breast self-examination process with you in her office, so that you could see for yourself exactly what is involved and she could check to see that you are applying the right amount of pressure for a thorough examination. Unfortunately, few doctors take the time for a careful training session, and the truth is, many of them may not be as expert in the procedure as you need them to be.

The steps we've just gone through should serve you well, but if you feel uncertain about performing them, try to go to a breast specialist to learn self-examination. Either the physician or a well-trained nurse at such offices will be able to get you started. The American Cancer Society provides free information on breast self-examination. Please consult the Resources at the back of the book for a list of some of these sources.

A Final—for the Moment—Word on Self-Examination

There is no way that we can statistically evaluate the benefits of breast self-examination, but we do know the following:
The procedure is simple.
It is free.
It can be done on a regular basis.
It is not dangerous.
It is the way most breast lumps are found.

PHYSICAL EXAMINATION BY A PHYSICIAN

If you are doing regular breast examinations of your own, why do you need a doctor's input, especially when the record of women finding breast lumps is so good?

The reason is that breast self-examination *plus* professional examination is even better. Research has shown that an annual physical examination of your breasts by a physician will improve your chances for successful treatment if you do get breast cancer because it will improve the chance of early detection. Even if there is nothing suspicious in your breasts, you should have an annual professional physical examination because a skilled doctor may find a lump you miss.

One of my patients came to me after her gynecologist, in a routine annual checkup, found a tiny lump that turned out to be a very early-stage cancer. The woman said, just before we performed a lumpectomy (see pages 117–120), "I'm glad you've drawn a line on my breast where you're going to operate. It's the first time I've been able to feel the lump myself."

Why does this happen?

Experience

The abnormality may be so tiny or ill-defined that only someone with a great deal of experience can feel it. Almost every day of my own life I examine women and feel certain tissue alterations. I think: "There's a lump." "Here's a thickening." "This spot feels different." "There's an asymmetry here." "Here's a place that's a little harder than the rest of the breast."

When a breast surgeon, in particular, feels a lump or a firm area, he is much more likely than a layperson to know what's going on, to be able to predict with a fair amount of accuracy the significance of any abnormality. Over the years, experience has taught breast surgeons how to interpret what we are feeling, because, over those same years, the findings from biopsies have illuminated what we've discerned during palpation. Many, many times, we have felt a lump, removed it in a biopsy, and then have learned, firsthand and from the pathologist's examination, what it was. It is not surprising, therefore, that breast specialists can tell so much by palpation.

Mammography

A **mammogram** is an X ray of the breast, taken with special equipment, which pictures the fat, the fibrous tissues, the lobes, the ducts, the blood vessels, and the other tissues of the breast. Mammography is performed by a radiologist or by an X-ray technician under the supervision of a radiologist. The interpretation of the mammogram is performed by a radiologist.

During a mammography, an X-ray beam is passed through the breast to produce a black-and-white negative picture called a film-screen mammogram. Like other "flat" pictures—paintings, maps, ordinary photographs—the mammogram gives us a two-dimensional view of a three-dimensional object.

No other method approaches the sensitivity of mammography in detecting the earliest and most curable tumors. Only the mammogram can pick up other important abnormalities such as microcalcifications. (See page 77.)

WHEN SHOULD I HAVE A MAMMOGRAM?

Guidelines for a mammography schedule differ depending on the purposes for which it is used and how various risks and benefits are interpreted. Mammography is used for **screening,** to monitor the breasts of apparently healthy women to make sure no abnormalities are present. It is also used for **diagnosis,** to investigate a lump or other problem of the breast.

The following list reflects my own views of a mammography schedule that is best for all women:

1. If a lump has been found during self-examination or by a physician, the next step in the investigation is a mammogram, whether or not the patient has had one in the preceding year.

2. Younger women who are symptom-free but who have a very strong family history of breast cancer (see page 243)

57

should start having annual mammograms at an age ten years earlier than that of the youngest first-degree relative to have breast cancer.

3. All women over forty—whether or not they are symptom-free—should have a mammogram every year.

4. All women, whatever their age, who have had *any* type of breast cancer should have an annual mammogram.

WHERE DO I GO FOR A MAMMOGRAM?

This is a particularly important consideration since the following factors can vary tremendously, depending on who does the X ray: the quality of the picture itself, the accuracy with which it is interpreted, the comfort of the patient during the procedure.

In Chapter Two, we discussed some of the methods you can use to find a good doctor. Review those again before you go for your mammogram. Bear in mind that mammography is one of the instances talked about earlier where, if there is not an excellent facility and an excellent radiologist nearby, you may want to go out of your community to find them.

The American Cancer Society (1-800-ACS-2345) can give you referrals to accredited mammographers in your community. Referrals are available, as well, from local divisions and units of the American Cancer Society. You can also call the National Cancer Institute's Cancer Information Service at 1-800-4-CANCER for the names of mammography providers in your area whose equipment and training meet the standards of the American College of Radiology.

Most important: Under the Mammography Quality Standards Act of 1992, all mammography facilities must be certified by the Food and Drug Administration. In most states, the accreditation that is the basis for the government certification is provided by the American College of Radiology, which takes into account the quality of the machine as well as the training and experience of the radiologist, who must submit samples of mammograms of several different types of tissue and other evidence of the quality of his X rays as well as of his interpretations. Most mammography facilities in the United States have been certified as of this writing. If no certificate has been issued, do not use the facility for your mammogram.

That is, I know, advice that may cause you problems and inconvenience, but nothing like the problems that can arise from using a substandard mammography facility.

There is one peculiar but valuable test of whether you are making a good decision: if a radiologist's office is not busy, if you can walk right in and not wait . . . probably you'd do best to walk right out again. The ironic fact is that though it can be annoying to have to wait for an appointment and then wait in a doctor's office, heavy traffic is almost inevitable in an excellent mammographer's office.

Also consider the following factors that are specific to this test:

1. Find out whether the doctor you are considering is a general radiologist or whether she specializes in mammography. You want someone who is an expert in this field.

2. Ask what mammography technique she uses. Film-screen mammography (see page 57) is the most accurate method of breast X ray now available and it requires the most sophisticated equipment. If, by some slim chance, you end up in the office of someone who uses a general X-ray machine, or uses xeromammography (see page 68) or any other equipment for mammography, do not have your breasts X-rayed there. Period.

3. Mammography studies are not easy to read. They should be interpreted by skilled, specifically trained, experienced specialists. One way to identify such experts is to ask the advice of a breast surgeon. Surgeons are in a good position to make this judgment, because they must rely on mammographers for specific information on such things as the precise location of the tumor, its shape, and its probable nature. If the person who performs and interprets the mammogram makes a mistake, the surgeon will know it all too soon and his own job will be a lot harder. It is crucial to good surgeons that they work with good mammographers. Use that fact to help yourself.

4. Mammography studies are done in several kinds of facilities by several different kinds of doctors and technologists.

A radiologist's office may only do mammography; or it may be a general radiology office where one radiologist has a special expertise in mammography. Mammography may also be done in a breast screening center, in a hospital, or in a physician's group practice.

Whichever of these you are considering, the basic questions to ask are

- Who is taking the picture?
- Who is interpreting it?
- Who is controlling the quality of equipment, technique, and the "reading" of the results?

Do not have a mammogram in the office of a gynecologist, surgeon, or internist who has a mammography machine on his premises and either "sends out" for interpretation or attempts to interpret on his own.

5. Mammograms vary in price but they tend to be expensive. Some insurance policies will cover only diagnostic mammograms. Others will pay for screening mammograms as well. In fact, the majority of states now require that health insurance policies cover screening mammograms; and certain communities, like Nassau County in New York, will provide screening mammograms free of charge to people who are unable to pay.

   There are centers around the country that will provide mammograms to women who need them on the basis of what they can afford to pay. Call the American Cancer Society at 1-800-ACS-2345, a local division or unit of the society, or the National Cancer Institute's Information Service at 1-800-4-CANCER for help in finding such a facility. You can also look for a community women's health center in the phone book, or ask your company's nurse or your local health department if they know where you can get a good screening mammogram you can afford.

It is important to stress that the recommended schedule of mammography we have just reviewed *should* be available to all women. Mammograms cost anywhere from fifty dollars to two hundred dollars, and the sad fact is that there are few communities that offer mammography screening to women who cannot afford it. Currently, Medicare pays only for mammograms every second year for women over sixty-five.

There is no doubt in my mind that this situation must change and that local, state, and federal governments must make it possible for women of all economic groups to have mammograms on the schedule we have outlined. Communities must also let women know how important regular mammograms can be to their health. In the long run, this will be of economic as well as social value.

HOW IS A MAMMOGRAM DONE?

1. You will be asked to remove all clothing from the waist up and any necklaces or jewelry you may be wearing. For this reason, you may find it more convenient to go for this procedure wearing a skirt or pants and a top.

   You should be given a paper gown or a clean cloth gown to wear when you walk from the place you change your clothes to the room in which the mammography machine is located. Fasten the gown front or back, however you are instructed.

   You will have to take the gown off before the actual picture is taken, and you will almost certainly find that the mammography room is quite cool; because the machines are computerized, a relatively cool temperature is required. Ask to keep your gown on until everything is ready, and if the operator is called out of the room before that time, ask for the gown back until the actual procedure is about to take place.

2. The machine that is used for mammography is a vertical structure. That means that you do not have to lie down for this X ray. Instead, you will stand or sit on a chair, and will be helped to prop your breast on the small protruding platform, first facing front and then to the side.

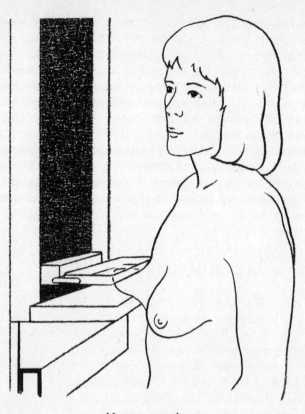

Mammography

You will be asked to lean forward and to raise your arms to very specific positions so as to open a clear view of the breast. The machine will then be adjusted so that your breast is firmly squeezed between two metal plates. An X-ray plate is inserted under your breast for the first pictures, then at its side for the next. You will be asked to stay perfectly still and to hold your breath while the picture is taken. The procedure is then repeated for the second breast.

3. The mammogram is read by the radiologist, and a report is sent to the physician who requested the study or to the physician you designate. This usually takes only a day or two.

WHOM WILL I DEAL WITH?

You should be seen by the radiologist before the X ray is taken. Though this is not universal practice, it is very important that the radiologist examine you in advance so that she herself will have seen any visible or palpable abnormality. Make sure to tell her the reason you have come for a test at this time and whether you know of any abnormality.

Several women have told me that they ask the person scheduling appointments whether the radiologist will be in the office at the time of their mammogram. They arrange for the test at a time when the radiologist will be present and able to see them.

You have come to the mammography facility either because there is some cause for concern or because you want to make sure there isn't. In both situations, the radiologist whose office it is owes you the courtesy and comfort of her attention.

In most facilities, under most circumstances, the actual X-ray pictures will be taken by an X-ray technologist.

When the pictures have been taken, the radiologist should have a preliminary look at them *before* you leave the office. If something unusual is seen in one view of the breast, for example, further X rays may be advisable. If this happens at a screening center, you may have to go elsewhere for further investigation, since only standard views are routinely taken.

Another reason it is important that the radiologist review the mammograms before you leave is to make certain that their quality is satisfactory. Occasionally that is not the case and more pictures are needed. It is unfair to the patient, and needlessly worrisome, to send her home and then call her back for a return visit (perhaps with the excuse that "follow-up" is needed) because the radiologist did not check the X rays at the time.

You should speak to the radiologist before you leave the office and discuss what has been found. Because the radiologist doesn't know you, she may prefer to give the full report to the physician, but you should be told whether the study is normal or needs further investigation, and when your own doctor will receive the report.

In fact, more and more radiologists are becoming involved in the diagnostic process, using various types of refined equipment and techniques to perform procedures such as biopsies as well as other investigations.

DOES A MAMMOGRAM HURT?

Though newer equipment requires less pressure than was formerly necessary, compression of the breast is necessary in order to get a good picture. This is bound to be a little uncomfortable, but what I have concluded from conversations with hundreds of patients is that none of it is really painful. None of it is more than mildly uncomfortable. It takes only a few minutes for the whole procedure.

That is not to say that you should grin and bear whatever comes your way. If you feel that a technologist is being especially rough or careless, ask her to stop at once and tell her you want to see the radiologist. If it's the radiologist who is conducting the examination, tell her the problem and ask her to be more gentle. Discuss the situation later with the physician who referred you and consider going elsewhere next time. If, for valid reasons, that is not an option, ask your referring doctor to talk to the radiologist about your discomfort.

WHAT ARE THE LIMITATIONS OF THE MAMMOGRAM?

Though mammography is the most sensitive tool for detecting early cancers, about ten to fifteen percent of the time a malignant lump will not show up on a mammogram. Why is that?

1. A mammogram only depicts the breast itself. There are areas close to the chest wall and at the periphery of the breast that do not actually show up on the film.

2. Even a slight shift in the position of the breast on the X-ray plate can mean that an abnormality is missed.

3. Mammograms, like other X rays, show soft tissue as gray. Hard or dense tissue appears as whitish. That means that the fat of the breast is gray on the mammogram; the lobes, the ducts, and other breast tissue are white. Tumors, because they are also dense, are white. For that reason, those in the dense or fibrous tissue of the breast are harder to spot—white against white—than tumors in

the fat—white against gray. Infiltrating lobular carcinomas are more likely than duct carcinomas to avoid detection because of the way they grow (see page 35).

Since the breasts of women of childbearing age are dense with the breast components needed for nursing, it may be somewhat harder to read their mammograms than those of older women whose breasts are primarily composed of fat and thus less dense.

4. An important caution is necessary here: even if the mammography report does not seem to indicate any abnormality, if you or your doctor has felt something unusual, or if you have the sense that something is not quite right in your breast, have a breast surgeon review the mammogram. He may have enough to make a diagnosis from these pictures or he may need more or better X rays.

A negative mammogram does not rule out the presence of cancer and a persistent lump should always be investigated. The track record of women and their physicians in detecting cancer is too strong to be ignored, even in the presence of a negative mammogram.

IS THERE ANY WAY TO MINIMIZE THESE LIMITATIONS?

Though there are limitations inherent in the technique, the best way to avoid problems in mammography is to go to an excellent radiologist in an excellent facility. Make sure the equipment has been certified by the Food and Drug Administration. Refer to the section above on choosing a radiologist and to the material in Chapter Two on choosing a physician.

If you know you may have a lump:

- Ask the doctor who has examined you to mark it with a spot or circle of ink before you go for your mammogram. (He should not use indelible ink for this purpose.)
- If for any reason that is not possible, make sure to explain to the person doing your mammogram that you are here because there is something suspicious in your breast. Show the responsible radiologist the place where you think it is.

- Whether or not it is marked, look for yourself; make sure that the area in question is positioned on the film plate. If you think it isn't, don't be shy about pointing that out. If it turns out you were wrong and the breast is, in fact, positioned properly—well, great! You've lost nothing.

IS A MAMMOGRAM DANGEROUS?

If there is something suspicious in your breast, the crucial thing is to find out what, if anything, is wrong. There is no significant radiation risk from investigative mammograms.

This question does arise, however, when we are considering this procedure for annual screening purposes. In that case, the most important reservation people have about mammography has to do with its safety. What is the risk that the exposure to radiation during the procedure—and from repeated mammograms over the years—will itself cause cancer?

The risk has been greatly reduced in recent years as mammography techniques have been improved. Much less exposure is now required than in the past. Strict guidelines are in place for the use of mammography equipment.

Still, you can't reduce the risk to zero. Anyone who tells you there is no risk is oversimplifying. Nevertheless, it is clear that, at this time, the benefits of mammography far outweigh its possible problems. There are several compelling reasons for this belief:

- Mammography is, at this time, the only tool we have to detect very early cancers.
- The probability of danger from radiation seems to be a great deal smaller than the probability of danger from an undetected cancer.
- The breast tissue of women in their teens and early twenties is more sensitive to low-level radiation than it is when they get older. For this reason, unless there are especially suspicious circumstances (see pages 57–58), we advise women under thirty-five not to have a mammogram.
- Conversely, we feel fairly confident that the radiation risk to women over thirty-five is very, very small.

At the moment, there are no known problems from high-quality mammography and it does seem to be doing a good job.

WHY IS MAMMOGRAPHY IMPORTANT?

Mammography is essential as a diagnostic tool if there is any abnormality of the breast. It is also the *only* screening tool for finding early cancers in seemingly healthy women.

When an annual mammogram is combined with physical examination by a doctor, there is more than a one-third reduction in mortality from breast cancer. We have established this figure on the basis of an almost-thirty-year ongoing random study of the incidence of breast cancer among a population of about 62,000 women, some of whom had regular mammograms and physical exams, others who did not. The data from this screening project by the Health Insurance Plan (HIP) of Greater New York have been confirmed in a variety of ways in other studies in the United States, Sweden, Holland, Denmark, and England.

When we combine mammography with professional physical examination and self-examination, we have a powerful early-warning system against breast cancer. And the earlier cancers are found, the better the chance for survival and for breast preservation.

Thermography

Thermography is a procedure that uses a special camera to measure and record the heat pattern of the breast, on the premise that tumors emit more heat than the normal surrounding tissue. Though this method has been used and investigated for over thirty years, clinical trials thus far have not demonstrated its effectiveness in detecting early breast cancer. There is no reason to undergo this examination unless you're willingly participating in an experimental study. (Nor is there any reason to wear a bra with a built-in heat-measuring device as a form of self-examination. Stick to the palpation techniques for self-examination we've already discussed.)

Transillumination

Sometimes called diaphanography, transillumination is based on the observation that cancerous tissue absorbs more infrared radiation than benign tissue. The breast is lit—"trans-illuminated"—and its image recorded on special film or, through another process, viewed on a television monitor. There is no reliable evidence that transillumination is useful in detecting breast cancer.

Xeromammography

A technique developed by the Xerox company, xeromammography is a form of mammographic examination that results in a blue image on white paper, a "positive" rather than a negative image. Although a few respected physicians use this technique, at this writing it does not appear to approach a mammogram in accuracy and refinement and the machine is no longer being manufactured.

Sonography

Also called ultrasound (and used during pregnancy to view the fetus), sonography uses high-frequency sound waves to examine the breast. The breast is covered with a jelly, and a small instrument called a transducer is slid across its surface. The transducer emits short pulses that either pass through the tissue or—if the tissue is solid—bounce back. The results of this sound-wave exploration are recorded on a screen and photographed. No radiation is used.

Because it cannot find microcalcifications or very small tumors, sonography is not a good screening tool. It is, however, very useful for studying a specific density previously seen on a mammogram. If the density is a liquid-filled cyst, the sound waves will go through it. If it is a solid lump—a fibroadenoma (see page 44) or a cancer—the sound waves will bounce back. Using the sonogram for guidance, the radiologist can also aspirate the cyst or obtain tissue from a solid mass for analysis (see pages 71–72).

CAT Scan

Computerized axial tomography (CAT or CT scan) uses radiation to create cross-sectional pictures that are combined to create extremely detailed images. They are valuable in distinguishing the density of tissue in many parts of the body and are therefore used extensively for medical diagnoses. We are not yet sure that CAT scanning is an effective method of examining the breast. It is expensive; it employs more radiation than mammography, and it sometimes requires the use of an intravenous contrast material that may entail some risks. At this time it is rarely used, except experimentally, to study the breast.

MRI

Magnetic resonance imaging (MRI) of the breast is now in its early stages, though it is used frequently in diagnosing conditions in other parts of the body. An image is created with the use of a magnetic field rather than with radiation. At this writing, MRI remains an experimental procedure for picturing the breast.

BIOPSY

What Is It?

Biopsy is a procedure that removes a sample of tissue from the body so that it can be examined under a microscope. In a breast biopsy, a tumor and surrounding tissue are removed and examined under a microscope so that the pathologist can identify the cells that are present, characterize them, and determine whether they are malignant. The details of the pathologist's examination can be found in Chapter Five.

Even the word *biopsy* can have frightening associations for many patients. For that reason, it is important to bear one fact in mind: most biopsies of breast lumps reveal no malignancy. For most women, therefore, biopsy is a reliable tool for establishing that they do *not* have cancer.

Why Do I Need a Biopsy?

As we've discussed before, an experienced doctor often knows by its "feel" what a lump is, and after a mammogram, he may be able to quite accurately predict whether a tumor or thickening in the breast is malignant or not.

That educated hunch, however, is not enough to go on. The final diagnosis of breast cancer depends on an examination of the suspicious tissue under a microscope.

Who Performs Biopsies?

Depending on the nature of the biopsy, the procedure should be performed by a surgeon or radiologist who is experienced in breast cancer diagnosis. The tissue that is removed during the biopsy is examined by a pathologist, a physician who specializes in identifying disease by microscopic examination.

What Are the Types of Biopsy?

Several kinds of biopsy are used to examine breast tissue. They are called fine-needle aspiration, core biopsy, and two forms of formal (open) biopsy: incisional biopsy and excisional biopsy.

FINE-NEEDLE ASPIRATION (FNA)

WHERE?

The procedure is usually done in the office of a surgeon or radiologist.

HOW?

The skin around the lump or thickening is cleaned with an antiseptic solution, usually alcohol or Betadine. A small amount of local anesthetic is injected into the skin. A fine, hollow needle, often called a skinny needle, is inserted into the lump and any fluid that is present is drawn into a syringe.

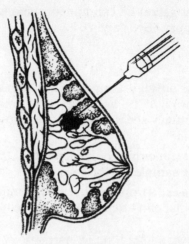

Fine-needle aspiration

If the lump is a solid (not fluid-filled) mass, we push the needle back and forth through the tissue to free some cells, aspirate them into the syringe, and then smear them on a glass slide. The slide is then treated with a preservative and sent to a laboratory for microscopic analysis by a pathologist.

PAIN?

Aspiration may be a little uncomfortable, but it should not cause you any serious pain. Most of the nerves of the breast are in the skin, which has been anesthetized.

FINDINGS

If the lump is a cyst, as breast masses most often are, needle aspiration turns out to be the treatment as well as the diagnosis. When the doctor withdraws the fluid, he not only identifies what's wrong, he also cures it.

When the fine-needle aspiration reveals a solid mass, and the sample is sent for analysis, a pathologist's report of "no malignant cells seen" does not necessarily mean that no cancer is present. It may mean only that this particular attempt to find a malignancy was unsuccessful. This result *always* requires that further investigation be conducted, usually by an incisional or excisional biopsy. (See page 76.)

LIMITATIONS

- When we are aspirating from a solid mass, the needle has to pass through the skin, fat, and breast tissue. Since we can't actually see it, there is the chance that we may miss the tumor.
- A breast tumor may be so dense that the needle is unable to dislodge samples of the cells.
- Even if a cell sample is obtained, it may be so small that the pathologist can't depend on it for reliable answers.

WHY BOTHER WITH FINE-NEEDLE ASPIRATION?

Even though the results of this procedure sometimes mean only that a surgical biopsy is needed, there are several circumstances in which a fine-needle aspiration is particularly helpful:

- When we have strong reason to suspect a malignancy, the aspiration may confirm the cancer's presence and no formal surgical biopsy will be needed.
- When several areas in the breast need to be evaluated.
- When we are sure there is a malignancy and that a mastectomy will be needed, we will often know from the aspiration what kind of cells we are dealing with and we will be able to skip the step of a formal biopsy (see pages 75–80) to provide that information.
- It is much less expensive than an operation and can be done at the time of mammography.
- And, best of all, needle aspiration is a wonderful method if it yields the happy ending that there was a cyst that now is gone.

CORE BIOPSY

WHERE?

This procedure is done in the surgeon's or radiologist's office.

How?

The skin is cleaned, usually with an antiseptic solution called Betadine, and a local anesthetic is injected.

A large-caliber needle is inserted into the lump to obtain a sliver of tissue, which is then sent to a laboratory for microscopic examination.

PAIN?

Because the needle is large and more manipulation is required, even though you have been given a local anesthetic, you may feel pain. If you do, immediately tell the doctor and ask for more anesthetic.

FINDINGS

Because actual tissue is removed with the core biopsy, more detailed information can be obtained than with a fine-needle aspiration biopsy.

LIMITATIONS

- Though the cell sample is larger than the one we get with needle aspiration, it is still quite small. Therefore, if cancer or a benign abnormality is not found, we still have to investigate further with a formal biopsy.
- When a well-defined, solid mass is present, highly accurate information can be obtained, permitting diagnoses of benign or malignant conditions to be made. However, with more subtle and less distinct "thickenings" of the breast, the sampling may be incomplete and a formal biopsy may still be needed even if no evidence of malignancy is found.

WHY BOTHER?

The larger sample obtained by core biopsy permits the pathologist to view suspicious cells in the setting of normal breast structures from which they may arise.

STEREOTAXIC BIOPSY

WHERE?

The procedure is carried out in a radiologist's office or in the radiology department of a hospital.

How?

It is performed in a sitting position or lying down prone on a specialized table. After a mammogram is taken, a needle is placed directly into the lump being tested with the aid of a computer, and its position verified. Depending on the caliber of the needle, either a fine-needle aspiration or core biopsy is now done.

Pain?

Depending on the size of the needle, you may feel some pain despite having been given a local anesthetic. If you do, ask the doctor for more anesthetic.

Findings?

It is a highly accurate procedure.

Limitations:

- If microcalcifications need to be investigated, this procedure cannot be done if the area involved is too tiny.
- When used to diagnose very small tumors, a stereotaxic biopsy may not provide us with a large enough sample to make it possible to tell the difference between premalignant changes and true cancers.

Why Bother?

This procedure is needed when a lump is seen in a mammogram but cannot be felt.

- If the tumor is benign, it may be possible to avoid a formal open biopsy.
- If the tumor is malignant, it may be possible to carry out a one-stage instead of a two-stage procedure (see page 79).
- It is much less expensive than a surgical biopsy and takes little more time than a mammogram.

SONOGRAPHIC BIOPSIES

Sonography may also be used to guide a small needle into a solid mass in order to remove cells. This procedure is called a fine-needle aspiration biopsy under ultrasound guidance. Similarly, a core biopsy can be performed under ultrasound guidance.

FORMAL (OPEN) BIOPSY

WHERE ARE FORMAL BIOPSIES DONE?

These procedures should always be performed by a surgeon in a facility where the tissue can be examined by a pathologist as soon as it is removed. This is only possible in a hospital or in an ambulatory facility with an excellent laboratory and a pathologist on the premises prepared to handle the tissue. If a surgeon insists that he can just as well do a biopsy in his office, unless the office is right in a hospital, you should go to someone else.

Biopsies are performed on an outpatient basis. You are not assigned a room or a bed; you do not have to stay overnight. The hospital department is often called the ambulatory center, or the day surgery. You should call your insurance company in advance to request authorization for the biopsy. Ask whether your policy requires a second opinion.

When you get to the facility, you will be asked to fill out forms that give personal, medical, and insurance information. You will be assigned a hospital identification number if you have not been a patient in this institution before. The admitting officer may fasten a plastic identification bracelet to your wrist.

Next you will be asked to change into a hospital gown. A nurse will interview you, as will the anesthesiologist, who may start an intravenous injection now or may wait until you get to the operating room. If the anesthesia has already been started, you will be wheeled to the operating room on a stretcher. Otherwise you will walk to the operating room where the anesthesia will be administered and the biopsy performed.

After the biopsy, you will be wheeled to a recovery room where your condition will be monitored by a nurse. When you are fully awake, you will be given something to eat, and then you are free to change back into your street clothes and leave. You should plan to have someone pick you up and take you home.

HOW?

A cut or incision is made in the skin to the depth necessary to reveal the suspected tissue. This is called an open or formal biopsy.

There are two basic types of open biopsy:

- If a tumor is large and only a small piece of it is removed for examination, the surgery is called an **incisional biopsy.**
- If a tumor is small and the biopsy actually removes it completely, the surgery is called an **excisional biopsy.**

Much of the surgical procedure is the same for both types of biopsy:

1. The surgeon will scrub his hands and will put on sterile gown, gloves, cap, and mask.
2. The skin of the affected breast is cleaned, usually with the antiseptic Betadine.
3. The upper part of the patient's body is covered with a sterile drape, except for the breast that is to be biopsied. Part of this drape separates the patient's head from the site of the surgery. As a result, the patient is not able to watch the procedure.
4. Because an electrical instrument called a cautery may be used (see below), a grounding pad is placed under the buttocks.
5. Anesthesia is then administered.
6. A cut is made in the skin over the tumor. The cut goes through the fat and breast tissue until the tumor is reached.
7. The surrounding tissue is spread apart so that the surgeon can get a clear view and full access to the tumor. In an incisional biopsy, a segment of the tumor is cut out; in an excisional biopsy, the entire tumor is removed.
8. To control bleeding, the surgeon may use a cautery and/or clamps or sutures.
9. When the tumor or segment has been removed, the surgeon stitches the tissue, the fat, and the skin to close the incision and then carefully bandages the site of the biopsy.

Needle localization

The sophistication of mammography technique alerts us to the presence of tiny tumors, some of which it may not be possible to see or feel without X ray. Most of these tumors turn out to be benign, but they do have to be removed for microscopic examination. To accomplish this, just before the surgery a technique called needle localization is employed:

1. Either in the hospital's radiology department or in her office, a radiologist X-rays the breast, locates the suspicious area, and inserts a needle into the breast so that its tip is at the site of the tumor. The needle has a tiny hook at its end that fixes it in place.
2. The patient immediately goes to the location where the biopsy will be performed and is prepared for surgery. The surgeon makes an incision and follows the needle's course to the site of the tumor.
3. The tumor is removed in a standard biopsy procedure.

Specimen radiography

Mammography may reveal the presence in the breast of **microcalcifications**, tiny flecks of calcium that sometimes can indicate the presence of an early breast cancer.

Microcalcifications are suspect if they are clustered in one area of the breast. In most instances, scattered specks of calcium are no problem. Microcalcifications ought to be investigated by biopsy—even though they are often harmless—if they are clustered or if they have appeared since the last mammogram. In fact, at present, among the most common reasons for biopsies is to investigate microcalcifications.

The problem is that though the microcalcifications are being picked up by the mammogram, we are not necessarily able to see them during surgery. Under these circumstances we probably have to take out a larger section of breast tissue than we would if there were a visible tumor. Therefore:

• We use needle localization to indicate the questionable area.
• We X-ray the excised section before the surgery is complete to make absolutely sure that we've adequately removed the tissue containing the calcifications.
• Both the X rays and the tissue are sent to the pathologist.

Anesthesia

Any time one makes a cut in the body, an anesthetic is needed to eliminate pain. Generally speaking, the type of anesthesia—as well as the type of biopsy—is determined by the size and location of the tumor.

- If the tumor or other abnormality is small, well-defined, and near the skin's surface, the surgeon will probably use local anesthesia, a medication that is injected into the site of the procedure to make it insensible to pain. (Local anesthesia may also be used after the incision is closed to minimize postoperative discomfort.)

- The skin's surface will be cleaned, usually with the antiseptic Betadine. The anesthetic is then injected into the skin and into the tissues surrounding the tumor.

- You will be awake and able to respond, though there will be no sensation in the area that has been anesthetized. The surgeon will pinch the skin or touch you with a surgical instrument to make sure the anesthetic is working. If you feel anything, by all means tell him.

- In addition to the local anesthesia, you may be given an intravenous medication, one that is injected into a vein. It will further reduce the pain and will relax you or put you briefly to sleep.

- A general anesthetic is a medication, usually in the form of inhaled gas, that causes a loss of sensation and of consciousness. It may be used for a large excision, particularly where cancer is strongly suspected or where there are other circumstances—such as a small but deep tumor—that may result in the patient feeling some pain. Using this type of anesthesia allows the surgeon to excise enough tissue to get information, not only about the tumor, but also about the surrounding tissue, during the first procedure. Often this is not possible with local anesthesia.

- In addition, there may be circumstances when the patient herself, for personal reasons, does not want to be awake during the procedure.

Before the biopsy, make sure to carefully discuss with the surgeon what anesthetic he plans to use, what the alternatives are, and under what circumstances he may decide to administer

78

another drug during the course of the procedure. Talk it over thoroughly until you understand and are comfortable with the plan.

PAIN?

You should feel no serious pain during a biopsy. If you do, tell the surgeon at once so that he can remedy the situation. You may feel some sensation of the tugging of skin or tissue. Women say that this feels peculiar or unpleasant but that it does not hurt.

After the biopsy you may feel the mild discomfort that can occur when any cut or wound is healing. Most women don't seem to need much medication to deal with this discomfort.

ONE-STAGE OR TWO-STAGE PROCEDURES?

It used to be that before a patient had a breast biopsy, she was asked to sign a statement that gave the surgeon permission to perform a mastectomy if he found cancer. This was based in part on the erroneous theory that introducing a needle or other instrument into the tumor or operating a second time would "spread" the cancer. Often, therefore, a woman could go in for a biopsy and wake up to find she'd had a radical mastectomy.

Women's advocacy groups very properly worked to eliminate this often traumatic surrender of control. The result is that the one-stage procedure has almost been eliminated. Most patients now have a biopsy, wait for the results, and then, if cancer is found, give themselves time to get used to the idea. The biopsy will provide the information necessary to explore treatment options with the surgeon as well as with other specialists. The definitive breast surgery is usually done later.

There are, however, some circumstances in which this "rule" of the two-stage procedure doesn't serve the patient best. In such instances, and with her understanding and consent, the biopsy and the surgery are performed in the course of the same operation:

- Some patients are adamant about wanting a mastectomy. They may not want to face two separate procedures or they may have a strong family history of breast cancer with close relatives who have died.

- The cancer may have been found at a stage when breast conservation is no longer feasible, and a one-stage procedure will spare the patient the ordeal of two separate procedures.

- Similarly, where breast cancer is strongly suspected, the patient and the doctor may have thoroughly discussed in advance breast conservation through a wide-excision removal of the tumor and surrounding tissue (lumpectomy), as well as the lymph nodes. In such instances, unless there are unanticipated findings, many women prefer to have the biopsy and surgery done in one stage.

You should review the biopsy plans carefully with your surgeon before the procedure and jointly arrive at a plan for your biopsy and any surgery that subsequently may be necessary. Also check with your insurance company to make sure that a second opinion is not required before a one-stage procedure.

RESULTS

We will discuss in the following chapter the procedure the pathologist follows to examine the tissue that has been surgically removed from the breast. We will also review the points the pathologist's report will cover. It is these, of course, that tell us definitively whether or not cancer cells are present.

If you are going to have a biopsy with a local anesthetic, it is a good idea to make a pact with your surgeon beforehand that even though you will be awake, you won't ask him while the procedure is taking place—and he won't tell you—how things look to him or what he thinks the percentages are. In fact, most of the time he doesn't really know, nor is it finally in your own best interests to distract him during the procedure. He is busy and needs to give his full attention to the surgery.

Hard though it is to wait for the results, it is worse to be given information that turns out to be inaccurate, or to receive important news while you are on the operating table under partial sedation and not really alert. It isn't until the pathologist's report on the frozen section is available (see page 83) that the results can be certain.

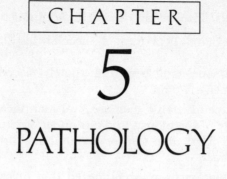

CHAPTER

5

PATHOLOGY

T he pathologist, the medical specialist who examines and analyzes the tissue removed during the biopsy, provides the key not only to finding out whether cancer is present, but also to the subsequent treatment. We have been more successful in helping people with breast cancer in recent years largely because we've been able to better tailor the treatment specifically to what the pathologist has discovered.

In the following sections we will look at how the pathologist works and how he arrives at his conclusions. It is not possible for the nonspecialist to absorb all the technical details of a pathologist's report, but some understanding of the process may help you to understand what your physician tells you after the biopsy, and may also help you to formulate important questions about the treatment that will be planned if cancer is found.

LABELING AND TRANSPORTING THE SPECIMEN

As soon as the biopsy is performed, the following steps are taken:

1. Each tissue sample is immediately placed in a plastic container.

2. The patient's name, her hospital identification number, the date of the biopsy, and a number or letter designated for the particular sample are marked directly on each container.

3. A requisition form is completed that gives the patient's name, the surgeon's name, specific details about the tumor and the specimen, a summary of the patient's related medical history, and a list of all the tissue samples that have been submitted.

4. The specimen containers, together with the form, are carried by an orderly or sent through a pneumatic tube carrier directly from the operating room to the pathology department.

5. In most hospitals, the pathology department has a direct intercom connection with the operating room. This is especially important if a quick, preliminary examination, called a frozen section (see below), is required by the surgeon before he completes the surgery.

Patients sometimes worry that there will be a mix-up and that the tissue the pathologist examines and reports on will not really be theirs. It is impossible to say, "No way. That could never happen." On the other hand, there are so many controls and identifying safeguards along the way that the chances of a mistake of this sort at a reputable hospital are practically nil.

THE PATHOLOGIST'S EXAMINATION AND REPORT

When the specimen arrives at the pathology laboratory, the process of examination immediately begins. The date and time the specimen arrives are recorded, a pathology number is assigned, and government-required formal documents are filled out to en-sure that specimens are properly identified. All this information is usually entered into a computer.

1. The pathologist first performs a *gross examination*, in which he reads the description on the pathology requisi-tion of each specimen he receives, and then inspects and notes on his report its physical characteristics, including weight, dimensions (width, height, and breadth), con-tour and shape, and texture. The pathologist may also comment on the specimen's color. (The fat of the breast is yellow, the ducts and other vessels are white. When a malignancy is visible to the eye, it may appear as an irregular patch of white discoloration.)

2. The specimen will next be cut, or *sectioned*, first for the *frozen section*, then for the *permanent section*. In prepa-ration for cutting, the specimen is coated with indelible ink so that the pathologist will always be able to identify the specimen's outer surface or margin.

3. A sample is taken from a few areas of the tumor or sus-picious tissue, as well as from the edges of the total speci-men, referred to as the margin.

4. A frozen section may then be performed. The results of this examination will be available in a matter of a few minutes.

   • A very small piece is cut from the excised tissue and a chemical is used to instantly harden or fix it. This hard-ened tissue is called a frozen section.

5. A permanent section is then prepared. It will take several days for the results to be obtained. The tissue that re-mains after the frozen section is placed in a preservative called formalin that fixes it in much the same way that boiling an egg hardens its contents.

6. Any water remaining in the tissue is removed and re-placed with paraffin.

7. After twenty-four hours the permanent section is firm enough to be prepared for microscopic analysis. Very

much the same analysis is done on the frozen section as well:

- The specimen is cut into slices that measure one fifty-thousandth of an inch, thinner than tissue paper, less than one cell thick.
- The slices are mounted on glass slides and stained with chemical dyes that will present different shades of red and blue when placed on different types of tissue.
- The pathologist then reads the slides under his microscope and issues a report on what he sees.
- Additional preserved tissue is carefully stored so that if questions arise in the future, it can be referred to.

People sometimes ask why we bother with the time and trouble of a permanent section if we've already done a frozen section. We use a frozen section to see if we can get a quick answer. This is possible because the slides prepared from a frozen section can be just as accurate as those from a permanent section if there is a positive diagnosis of cancer.

The problem lies with the opposite result: if no cancer cells are found, we cannot be satisfied with the results of a frozen section. It is not as comprehensive as a permanent section.

- Since only a minute part of the tumor is taken for examination, we cannot be sure that the unanalyzed portion doesn't contain malignant cells.
- If the original tumor is quite small, we don't really want to "waste" tissue on a frozen section, since the results may not be definitive. We would rather use the complete specimen for the more reliable results of the permanent section.

What Does the Pathologist Observe?

THE CELLS

You may hear the terms *differentiated* or *undifferentiated* in reference to cancer cells. These terms describe the degree to which the cells seen under a microscope resemble normal cells.

Intraductal carcinoma

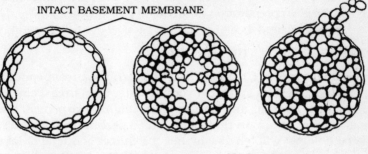

INTACT BASEMENT MEMBRANE

[1] Normal duct
1 to 2 layers of
normal cells.

[2] In situ *cancer*
Duct filled with
cancer cells.

[3] Invasive
(infiltrating)
ductal carcinoma
Cancer cells invade
through the basement
membrane into the fatty
tissue of the breast.

Differentiated cells are close to normal cells in appearance; undifferentiated cells have an abnormal appearance.

Normal ducts and lobules are lined around their periphery with a single or double layer of cells, arranged in an orderly pattern. When cancer develops, the proliferating cells present themselves not in orderly rows, but randomly dispersed, sometimes forming a complete blockage of the duct. This is an *in situ* cancer. If these cells break through the basement membrane of the duct or lobule, this is an invasive cancer.

Normal breast cells are under strict growth control and have a rigorously programmed, very limited ability to divide. Malignant cells grow and divide rapidly.

Normal cells have a dense central structure called the nucleus, which contains the chromosomes. The rest of the cell, called the cytoplasm, is primarily engaged in manufacturing proteins and processing glucose.

In normal cells, the genetic material DNA appears within two sets of chromosomes. This normal status is called *diploid*. Malignant cells have either fewer or more chromosomes, and are referred to as *aneuploid*. In a test called *flow cytometry*, performed after the microscopic examination, the pathologist examines the

DNA content of the cells to determine the number of chromosomes, as well as to see whether the tumor cells are manufacturing new DNA in preparation for division (the S phase).

THE LOCATION OF THE CANCER

As we discussed in Chapter Three, though the breast contains fat and blood vessels and other components, most breast cancers originate in the ducts and lobules. About eighty-five percent of all breast cancer occurs in the ducts, fifteen percent in the lobules. The pathologist will tell us whether the cancer is ductal or lobular.

The pathologist examines samples from the edge, or margin, of the piece of tissue that was removed during the biopsy in order to determine whether there is a clear border of normal tissue around the specimen. If there isn't, if the cancer goes right up to the inked edge, that may indicate that there may be more cancer in the adjacent tissue remaining in the breast.

The pathologist will examine the tumor and the surrounding tissue to see whether cancer is present in the fat of the breast, the blood vessels, or the lymphatics, or whether it is *in situ*—that is, confined to the original site.

He will note whether there is only one duct with an *in situ* cancer, more than one, or whether ducts throughout the specimen contain *in situ* cancers.

Once the cells have broken through the basement membrane of the duct or lobule, they invade or infiltrate the surrounding tissue. Depending on the site of origin, the pathologist will report whether the cancer is an infiltrating ductal carcinoma or an infiltrating lobular carcinoma.

(Remember that the lymph nodes in the armpit are not examined at this time. If there is a need for later breast surgery, the underarm lymph nodes will be removed and examined then. This procedure is discussed in the section on surgery, Chapter Seven.)

THE HORMONE RECEPTOR ASSAY

In addition to performing the gross and microscopic analyses of the tissue, before fixing the specimen the pathologist prepares the tissue for a hormone receptor assay, a test that measures the presence of estrogen and progesterone receptors in the tumor cells. Because this test takes time, the results will rarely be ready at the time of the pathologist's report on the permanent section, but will usually be available in about two weeks.

If these receptors are present, the tumor is said to be estrogen-receptor positive or progesterone-receptor positive. In fact, if there are two separate tumors in the same breast, when we examine them we may find that one is receptor-positive, the other negative. These findings have an impact on the planning of post-surgical treatment, since receptor-positive cells are more likely to respond to hormonal therapy.

The Final Diagnosis

The final pathology report is the place in which the pathologist summarizes his findings and establishes the diagnosis.

The final diagnosis may conclude that the condition is benign, in which case the patient is home free. Or it may identify the cancer cells, describe whether the cancer is infiltrating or confined, and state whether the cells are well-differentiated or undifferentiated. As we will see, these conclusions will help determine the course of treatment.

The pathology report may be available two or three days after the biopsy, though in some pathology departments it can take as long as a week. Before the biopsy, you should ask your surgeon how long the hospital laboratory usually takes to issue the pathology report. Having that information in advance will help make the waiting easier, since you will know that the amount of time is routine for this laboratory and not an indication that something is wrong or that information is being withheld.

THE MEANING OF THE DIAGNOSIS

If the pathologist's report concludes that only a benign condition is present, you can feel both relieved and reassured. You have had a physical examination, a mammogram, and a biopsy. You have done everything possible, with the very best techniques now available, to make sure there are no malignant cells present. That exercise wasn't a waste of time or money—it provided you with invaluable information.

If the biopsy reveals the presence of cancer, the pathologist's findings will help point the way to the best treatment. Yet the pathologist can describe only what has been removed from the breast and examined in the laboratory. What he has found is crucial, but it is not the whole story. His findings must be interpreted jointly with those of the surgeon who performed the biopsy and actually saw the tissue in its natural setting. If any uncertainty regarding the nature of the tumor remains, you or your surgeon may want to get a second pathologist's opinion on the findings.

The surgeon should share the pathologist's report with you and interpret for you its detailed findings and the treatment he recommends based on those findings. How you act on that information is the subject of the next chapter.

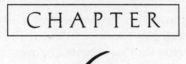

CHAPTER

6

AFTER THE
DIAGNOSIS

❧

There's almost no need to describe the relief and joy everyone feels when the news is good, when no malignancy is
found. One of my patients recently said, "Each day I
waited seemed like an eternity. I thought Tuesday would
never pass and then, even though I went to work on Wednesday,
the whole office seemed to be like a slowed-down movie projec-
tion. Then, when we found out—well, my boyfriend and I were
both crying and laughing at the same time. There's no way to tell
you how I felt, as if I had entered real life again."

The story is obviously different when a malignancy is found.
This is a moment that for most people becomes frozen in time.
Women can recall the date and the exact circumstances under
which they heard the news that they had cancer. The scene is
etched vividly in their minds: they see where they were, hear the
voice and the words again and again.

89

It is information that does not go down easily. Patients who ordinarily have perfectly good memories call a few hours after they have learned that they have breast cancer to ask me to repeat what I said because "it did not sink in."

This is the most normal and human of reactions. It is very hard to absorb everything you are told under such circumstances. If you want to make such a telephone call, your doctor should be sympathetic and tell you again what you need to know.

THE PHYSICIAN'S ROLE

In many instances, the doctor who on the basis of a physical examination, a mammogram, or a pathologist's report is the first to say "I think it's cancer" can seem to the patient to be the villain. When the very person to whom you have turned for help becomes the bearer of horrible news, it is hard to imagine that that same human being can be your advocate, and it's easy to feel distrustful.

It is also true that women are sometimes upset about the way in which the news of their breast cancer was broken to them. Their complaints are often justified, but speaking as a doctor, I have to say that there is no good way to tell someone she has cancer. There is no good time or place to convey this news.

This is not a book whose theme is to explain how difficult life is for physicians. It is not "harder for me than it is for you," and I have little patience for physicians who equate their own strong feelings of sympathy with the real thing—the pain and shock their patients are experiencing. Nevertheless, having to tell a patient she has cancer is a very hard thing to do. The sadness and stress that are involved can take their toll on any compassionate person. Sometimes a doctor will draw back and seem to remove himself from the patient because he cannot cope with the powerful emotion of this encounter. Understandable though such an attitude may be, it is not what the patient needs at this moment when reassurance and clarity are required.

RECEIVING THE NEWS

All of us have our own ways of dealing with what we see as a threat to our lives, and that is how most people perceive a diagnosis of cancer. But there does seem to be a general pattern in these reactions: first we are shocked and frightened; then we confront the danger. We prepare ourselves to face it by completely focusing on the problem itself.

The first reaction of a woman in my office recently was to put her hand up protectively and say in an anguished voice, "Don't say that. Don't talk about it. There's no way it can happen to me."

Other women have a delayed reaction. They tune out and need to call or come back again to actually register what they have been told. Still others don't seem particularly distressed at the moment. They throw themselves into a conversation about treatment and prognosis and it is only later, usually on that same day, that the news really hits them.

AN APPROACH TO THE DIAGNOSIS

As a patient, you don't have any control over how you will be presented with the facts of your illness. But for me as a cancer specialist and for you as a cancer patient, there is an approach to the diagnosis that is most desirable and, ultimately, most beneficial, no matter how the diagnosis has been conveyed. Remember:

- Something *can* be done. This is a difficult problem, but it is possible to deal with it. A program can be devised that will help.
- Breast cancer is certainly not an illness one would choose to have, but it does respond to treatment.
- The most productive attitude for both the doctor and the patient is to approach the illness with a determined and optimistic pragmatism.

91

ACTING ON THE DIAGNOSIS

After the shock, faced with the knowledge that you have breast cancer, you have to be as smart as you can be.

First, consider again whether the doctor who has presented you with the diagnosis is the right one to continue taking care of you. Refer to the section on page 14 on finding and choosing a doctor. At this point, many insurance companies require a second opinion, before any further surgery. Even if your policy does not have that restriction, you should consider whether you want to seek that second opinion. (See Chapter Two.)

Find someone whose attitude, skill, and compassion allow him to say to you, verbally, or through his reputation and demeanor, "I care about you. I am here to help you. I can do it well. There is hope." You should feel, after your search, your consultation, and your deliberation, "You are the one I have decided to trust. I will participate in all decisions, but I want you to be my ombudsman, an expert with whom I can share the responsibility for evaluating and treating my illness."

If you cannot enter into a relationship with a doctor feeling confident about both those declarations, look elsewhere.

HOW FAST DO I HAVE TO ACT?

Some of the considerations here are psychological, some medically significant. Whichever factors you want to assess, you should move with all deliberate speed—but you should not, even at this point, rush into a hasty decision.

A sensible goal is to have treatment under way within three to four weeks after diagnosis. Is it dangerous to wait that long? The answer is straightforward: though growth rates for different types of breast cancer can vary, there is no evidence of a measurable change for any of them in a period of three or four weeks.

If you have selected a surgeon and then are told he cannot operate for a week or two, that is probably fine. Most surgeons will try to schedule your procedure as soon as possible. As with mammographers, excellent surgeons are bound to be busy, but it is almost certainly worth waiting a short time for a surgeon with both superior technical skill and sound judgment.

In fact, there is a tricky point to consider: if a breast specialist can take you right away, it is legitimate to wonder if he is busy enough to be the right person for you. Surgeons who have excellent track records, judgment, and experience are almost certain to have crowded schedules, and will rarely be able to operate immediately. Under most circumstances, they are also worth waiting for, not only because, in the language of our trade, they know "how to cut," they also know "what to cut."

Nonetheless, getting through the waiting period, or the period in which you are making your choices and decisions, can be very difficult. Some women rush to action. They want to get the whole thing over with, to get the cancer out of their bodies as quickly and thoroughly as possible.

Other women can get stuck in conflicting advice, getting so much information that they unnecessarily complicate what might otherwise be a fairly simple procedure. Reread Chapter Two now if you feel you need help in the process of selecting a surgeon. Read the material that follows, in Book II, in order to understand and evaluate the types of treatment that are being offered to you.

ALTERNATIVE TREATMENTS

When you go through Book II, you will notice that there is no chapter on what are popularly called alternative treatments for breast cancer. That is because I consider reliance on such treatments a prescription for tragedy. The only time I ever see what I call nineteenth-century cancers—those that are large and have spread extensively by the time of the first visit—is when a woman comes to me after being treated with unconventional treatments or when she has relied on the curing techniques of disciplines like Christian Science.

What we are seeing under such circumstances is a missed opportunity to cure a now-uncontrolled cancer. Standard treatment, as we will see, works to a very large degree. As far as my own and other research has shown, nontraditional treatments do *not* work. If they did, they would certainly be used by many doctors. I honestly do not believe it is the resistance of the medical establishment to unusual techniques that accounts for the fact that most physicians do not rely entirely on dietary or psychological or other unproven modes of treatment.

Physicians want to help people, both for their patients' sakes and for their own. And particularly when we are dealing with people with cancer, we are willing to stretch the boundaries of what may or may not help.

There is no harm in vitamin supplements, high-carbohydrate diets, et cetera, *unless* they delay, interfere with, or replace other proven treatments or cause health problems of their own. Good nutrition, especially when you are sick, is important for your well-being, but it is not a substitute for vigorous, effective treatment.

A patient with seriously advanced disease recently told me that she watched the tumor on her breast grow for several months because every time she mentioned it to the "alternative physician," he would tell her that the symptom was unimportant, that "local disease" was the last to respond to his treatment, and that the tumor growth was therefore of no significance!

In Chapter Fourteen, Prevention, we will discuss the question of psychological attitude and cancer. Rather, we will discuss my own strong feeling that you don't get cancer because of your psyche. To intimate that psychological attitude does play such a role increases unfairly the burden on people who are ill. It is the worst instance I know of laying a guilt trip on someone. The same may be said about treating breast cancer with psychological methods.

Certainly you should do everything you can to help yourself approach your illness in a positive, constructive way. You should do everything you can to make yourself feel comfortable emotionally. We don't know everything about the mysterious factors that govern why it is that one patient survives and another does not, under similar medical circumstances. We *do* know that imaging, enemas, macrobiotic diets, relaxation techniques, deep massage, group healing, and the like are *not* a substitute for good medical treatment.

94

YOUR PERSONAL ADVOCATE

Though we talked about this earlier, in Chapter Two, it is worth repeating what I think may be a crucial part of your treatment and recovery: the way to be a "good patient" is not to be a docile, obedient one.

Some interesting research has been done that seems to indicate that patients who take an active part in the management of their own illnesses—not just breast cancer—do better than those who passively accept what is prescribed for them. I know that the call to be an active participant in your own treatment can sound intimidating. There may, in fact, be times when you will be tired or discouraged or frightened, or simply need help in understanding what is being told to you.

"I've got a really good memory," one of my patients told me. "Part of my job is to store away in my brain all sorts of facts. But after I sat in your office that day and listened to you tell me about my cancer and what you recommended—well, by the time I got home, I couldn't remember anything. I couldn't tell my husband one clear fact—except that I had it."

- You need someone to help you remember.
- You need someone to help you evaluate what is being recommended.
- You need someone whose shoulder you can lean on.

If you have not already done so, by all means try to get yourself a personal advocate, someone who understands that you want his or her presence when you deal with breast cancer. For some women, that person will be their husband or partner. Other women, even if they are part of a couple, will feel that an adult child, or a sister or other relative or a friend, has the steadiness and sympathy and good sense they need.

And those *are* the qualities you want. Someone who has had breast cancer may be the right choice. Someone close to you who is a health worker or doctor may be suitable. But the main ingredients are these three: steadiness, sense, sympathy.

Talk directly to the person you choose. Don't assume, just because you ask him or her to accompany you to one doctor's visit or a test, that the person realizes you want a continued presence. Explain that you are not asking your advocate to make decisions for you and that you are not going to require a constant babysitter. Do spell out exactly what you have decided you're going to need:

- Do you want her to sit in with you during medical consultations?
- Do you want her to participate in conversations with the physicians you consult?
- Do you want her to meet with you before your appointments to help you formulate the questions you should ask?
- Do you want her to take notes?
- Is she someone who will understand if you change your mind? You may decide along the way that you prefer to proceed on your own, or to find a new person to help you. That is perfectly fine. Your first priority is to feel confident in what you are doing, as well as in the people who constitute your support system.

YOUR FEELINGS ABOUT YOUR DIAGNOSIS

Why Me?

At one time or another during our lives we have all heard the phrase "Why me?" and to a certain extent, at one time or another during our lives, we have all asked that question or shared the feeling it expresses. It is human nature to look around us and wonder why, out of all the people we know, this particular misfortune is being meted out to us.

We will talk in Chapter Fourteen about the scientific risk factors of any particular woman's getting breast cancer, but it is important to understand that the illness is not a punishment for bad or imprudent behavior. Escaping it is not a reward. Despite what you may have read in the popular press, *there is no such thing as a cancer personality.*

As to the philosophical question raised here, I think of the response of one of my patients who asked, "Why *not* me? So many women get breast cancer these days that it's no big surprise any one person gets hit with it."

In fact, after the initial reaction to a positive diagnosis, the question "Why me?" seems to disappear and most women get on with what they have to do to take care of themselves.

But I Feel Fine

One of the reasons the diagnosis of breast cancer comes as such a shock to many women is that usually they have no symptoms. They aren't short of breath, they don't have any pain, their kidneys are fine, their digestion. They may not even feel a lump. Many patients say they have "never felt better."

And yet they have been told that they have cancer, a grave disease. One woman, in trying to explain this dichotomy to me, held up a strand of her hair. She said, "It's as if someone told me that at the end of this piece of hair there is a knot that can kill me. I would find that very hard to believe because it isn't causing me the slightest trouble."

All I could think to tell her was that the best thing she could do, if that were the case, would be to get rid of the knot. And that—getting rid of the knot—is what we must turn to next: the treatment of breast cancer.

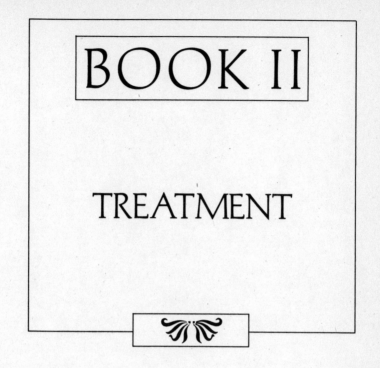

BOOK II

TREATMENT

CHAPTER

7

SURGERY

✥

Surgery is the first line of defense against most breast cancers, and for most patients it is the primary means by which a cure can be achieved.

That is not a new piece of information. Surgery—cutting the cancer out of the body—has been the basic treatment for many years. What has changed are the kinds of treatment that now supplement breast surgery and the kinds of surgery now performed.

It used to be thought that "the more the better"—the more tissue you removed, the better the chance of getting all traces of cancer and therefore preventing a recurrence. Because of what we have learned in recent years, less radical surgery has become common. At the present time, most women whose cancers are detected early can be treated without breast removal, with the excision of the cancerous lump, a margin of normal tissue, and the underarm lymph nodes, followed by treatment with radiation.

Twenty-five years ago radical mastectomy—an extensive procedure we will examine in the following pages—was the only treatment for breast cancer. When modified radical mastectomies became more common and a woman asked a surgeon about them, she might be told, "Sure, have a modified radical if you want to play Russian roulette with your life." When, several years later, lumpectomy—which is a partial mastectomy—was developed, that same surgeon might have told an inquiring patient, "Sure, have a lumpectomy if you want to play Russian roulette with your life."

There are people in all walks of life who like doing things the "same old way." They tend to stick with the ideas and methods they are familiar with. Don't choose such a person as your surgeon. Find a surgeon with good judgment, who is open to new ideas, and whose techniques are not limited to what *used to be* standard. To put it plainly, do not choose a surgeon who hasn't changed his ways in twenty years. You should be told all the options available to you.

The treatment of breast cancer is less standardized than that of many other illnesses. Because they know this, some patients believe that there are many different surgical procedures to choose among. In fact, there are only two:

- The breast is conserved in a procedure commonly known as lumpectomy; this is always followed by radiation therapy and sometimes by hormone and/or chemotherapy.

- The breast is removed in an operation called mastectomy. Breast reconstruction may be used after mastectomy, either immediately or at a later date, and systemic treatment may also be used.

These surgical procedures and the circumstances under which they are appropriate are described in the pages that follow. As you will see, making a decision about what kind of surgery is to be done depends on what seems correct for the pathology that was found, the size of the tumor and breast, as well as on what is acceptable to the patient.

BEFORE THE SURGERY

Drugs and Allergies

If you have been having any discomfort such as headaches and have been using any pain medication containing aspirin, you should stop taking it a week or two before surgery because aspirin may interfere with blood clotting. Before you go to the hospital, prepare a list of all medications you are taking, as well as the dosages, and take it with you to the hospital. Be precise in informing the resident or nurse who takes your medical history of these medications. If you have taken aspirin or any other prescription or over-the-counter drug in the last few days, mention it. Also be sure to tell the resident or nurse of any allergies you have, particularly to medications, even though your own physician may already have this information on record.

The use of monoamine oxidase inhibitors (MAOIs) such as Nardil or Parnate is particularly problematic, and these should be stopped two weeks before surgery. These are antidepressive medicines and you should check with your physician for possible temporary alternative therapy. It is advisable to stop drinking alcohol and smoking at least two weeks before surgery as well.

Hospital Arrangements

Someone in the surgeon's office will make arrangements with the hospital for your admittance, taking into account your needs as well as the availability of a bed, an operating room, and the anesthesiologist. You will probably be asked whether you want a private or semiprivate room, but the hospital often will not be able to accommodate your wishes because of overcrowding. Bear in mind that most hospital insurance covers only semiprivate rooms and that you will have to pay the difference in the daily rate if you choose a private room. Ask in advance what the prices are so that you won't be anxious about the cost during your hospital stay. You will usually be admitted the day of your surgery, several hours before the scheduled time of the operation.

Admission

Procedures for admission can differ a great deal from hospital to hospital, as do the amount of time you have to wait and the atmosphere of the admitting office. It is really a good idea, if it is possible, to have someone accompany you. You should also bring something to read or a crossword puzzle or anything else that will divert you in case there is a delay.

You will need your insurance card and any other health insurance or Medicare/Medicaid information that may be relevant. The hospital may clear your admission with your insurance carrier. You will be interviewed by an admissions officer and asked for the name of the person to be notified in case of an emergency.

Preadmission Testing

During the week before surgery you will have an appointment at the hospital for routine blood tests, an electrocardiogram, and a chest X ray. Additional studies such as a bone scan may be ordered at this time.

Your General Medical Condition

Because you will not be in the hospital for a medical workup, you should make sure that you report to the anesthesiologist and to the surgeon such matters as heart, lung, or circulatory disease; diabetes; or any other current medical condition you may have. Tell them if you have a cold or an upset stomach, or if you drink, smoke, or use drugs.

Don't dismiss any detail as too insignificant or embarrassing to mention. It is better for the medical team to be aware of all this information than to be surprised by some complication. If you are under the care of a cardiologist or internist, you should inform that doctor about your surgery. These specialists and your surgeon should communicate so that any appropriate care will be available if you need it.

Blood Transfusions

Blood transfusions are not used during biopsies or lumpectomies and are rarely needed during most mastectomies. Certain types of breast reconstruction, however, may require transfusion and you should therefore discuss the possibility with your physician and consider whether you want to donate blood yourself before your surgery to be stored so that it will be on hand should you need it. As far as we know, monitoring for the AIDS virus and other contamination of our stored blood supply is now effective; but many people are understandably concerned about this problem, especially given the gravity and extent of the AIDS epidemic. You can donate up to three units of blood at one-week intervals, and if there is enough lead time before your surgery, you may want to do that. As we have said, you probably won't need blood, but there is no harm in discussing the possibility of transfusion with your surgeon.

Talk to the Surgeon

You should have a clear understanding of what is going to be done, and the reasons for any particular procedure. You should also be aware of any risks of the surgery, which leads to a pre-surgery formality, the informed consent form, that many patients find quite troubling.

INFORMED CONSENT

The usual procedure is that after you have been admitted to the hospital, and before your surgery, you will be asked to sign an **informed consent** form. Your doctor or a staff resident with whom he works should present this form to you. It should be given to you prior to any sedation, which can affect your alertness, and enough in advance of the surgery for you to be able to read it carefully without feeling pressured. The form usually will specify:

- the name of the surgical procedure
- the doctor's name
- that the risks of the surgery and the anesthetic have been explained to you
- that intravenous medication, including drugs, anesthesia, and blood transfusions, may be administered
- that any tissue or parts that are removed during the surgery may be examined and disposed of
- that you understand all of the foregoing and that you consent

Some forms ask a lot more. They may ask for consent to videotaping or televising of the procedure. They may ask you to consent in advance should the surgeon decide, during the course of the operation, that other measures are necessary.

These forms are so broadly drawn because they were designed to cover many types of surgery. In abdominal surgery, for example, there is a strong possibility that unforeseen complications may arise. Breast surgery, on the other hand, is a fairly straightforward operation and there are rarely any complications.

If the procedure specified on the form has a different name than that which you and the surgeon agreed upon, ask that it be changed. It should very explicitly state the surgery you have consented to undergo. If there is anything else on the form that worries you, ask to see your doctor. Make sure you understand and feel comfortable with what you are signing. Cross out and initial anything you don't agree to. You should not be going into surgery worried about the fine print on a consent form. You might even want to ask your surgeon whether you can have the form to study a few days in advance so you can make sure you are comfortable with it.

Informed-consent forms were designed to make sure that doctors do tell patients precisely what is planned for them as well as the risks therefrom. The form obviously also protects the doctor, in that it spells out what he has told the patient he plans to do. In a sense, however, the form is less important than it looks. The physician is responsible for what he does, whatever the form says. And, from another perspective, the best insurance against mishap in surgery is not informed consent, but an excellent doctor.

A COMPANION

If you are going to have ambulatory surgery (see page 75), you are required to have someone with you to help you get home; but most people, whatever kind of surgery they are going to have, like to have a friend or relative with them after the operation. If you feel that way, tell your surgeon, and ask him to arrange with the hospital to allow that person to be in your room.

Ask in advance approximately how long it will take before you will be brought to your room after surgery. This estimate should include possible delays before the procedure and take account of the time of the surgery and the time afterward in the recovery room. Make a definite arrangement about when and where the surgeon will meet with your friend or relative to report on how the surgery went. After surgery, there is often needless confusion and anxiety for the family and the physician because they have trouble finding each other.

Remind your family or friends that the surgeon will be able to tell them whether the operation went well, whether there were any complications, and what your general condition is. Remember, however, that he will not be able to give them the kind of detailed information about your condition that will be available only after the pathologist's report, nor will he be able to say exactly how long you will be in the hospital or what the next step in your treatment will be.

Nursing

Many of my patients ask whether they should hire a private-duty nurse to be with them after the surgery. If you can afford it, or if your insurance covers the cost, do it. Make the arrangement before your surgery so that the nurse will be there when you are brought back to your room. Hospital nursing staffs are very lean in these economically difficult times, and your own nurse, for at least the first two shifts after your surgery, can be enormously helpful in such things as monitoring your blood pressure, giving you a bedpan or taking you to the bathroom, administering your medications, and keeping you comfortable. If your insurance company is reluctant to pay for private-duty nurses, ask your surgeon whether he can write a note explaining why such nursing is essential.

Private-duty nursing is very expensive, and if it is not possible for you to manage this cost, ask a competent friend or family member to stay with you, if possible, for the remainder of the day and night following your surgery.

Food and Drink

You will be instructed not to eat or drink anything after midnight of the night before the surgery is scheduled.

Other Preparations

Your armpit may be shaved in preparation for lymph-node dissection. (See pages 113–115.)

You will be asked to remove all jewelry (including watches, chains, and rings), as well as any eyeglasses, contact lenses, or dental bridges. Give these things to your companion to keep for you.

Because electrical instruments used during surgery may react with synthetic fabrics, any underpants you wear must be cotton.

GETTING READY FOR THE SURGERY

As we saw when we discussed surgical biopsy:

1. The surgeon will put on a scrub suit, cap, and mask. He will scrub his hands, put on sterile gloves, and be helped into a sterile gown.
2. The patient's skin in the area to be operated upon will be cleaned, usually with an antiseptic solution called Betadine.
3. The patient's body will be covered with a sterile drape, leaving uncovered only the area to be operated upon.

Monitoring Devices and Other Auxiliary Equipment

You will be very carefully watched all during the surgery.

- A cuff will be placed on your arm to measure your blood pressure.
- An electrocardiograph machine will monitor your heart rate.
- A clip will be placed on your fingertip to measure blood oxygen, and to monitor the conduct of the anesthesia.
- A tube may be placed in your throat to help you breathe.

- A grounding pad will be placed under your buttocks because an electric cautery may be used.

- Stockings that through compression prevent clotting will be placed on your lower legs.

- Sometimes, during an extended operation, a kind of boot may also be used to prevent clots from forming in your legs.

In sum, the latest technical equipment will be brought into play in the operating room to make the surgery as risk-free as possible. Much of this equipment will be hooked up while you're still awake, and there may be a fair amount of conversation going on among a fair number of men and women. There may also be a lot of noise of equipment being put into place.

Patients sometimes say that they felt as if they were being completely ignored during what one woman described as "all that frenzied activity." The fact is, people are getting ready for the surgery about to be performed and getting you ready to receive its benefits. That is what most of the bustle is about. It is, however, inexcusable for doctors, nurses, or technicians to alarm the patient by thoughtless comments. The anesthesiologist and the surgeon should take a few minutes to talk to you in as reassuring a manner as possible, but it is wise to remember that this is a very busy time for everyone in the operating room.

Anesthesia

An anesthesiologist is a specialist who, after receiving a medical degree, has gone on for several years of training in anesthesiology, the science of administering drugs that induce a loss of sensation and of consciousness.

The first thing to say about anesthesia is that you should meet the anesthesiologist yourself and talk to her, person to person, before your surgery.

- She should take your medical history and ask you, among other details, about any problems with the functioning of your heart, your lungs, or your circulation.

- Any allergies should be carefully reviewed, as well as any prior experiences with anesthesia.

• Tell the anesthesiologist anything you think may be relevant: if you have a cold, tell her. This is not a time for secrets. It's another chance to make sure that all the details of your condition are known. Remind the anesthesiologist if you are a heavy smoker or drink a lot or use drugs or other substances. If a nurse asks you the same questions, answer her as well. There's no harm in giving as much detail as you can and it is in your own interest to be frank.

The type of surgery as well as the patient's medical history determine what anesthesia will be used. However, since breast surgery is a fairly superficial procedure, on the "outside" of the body, it does not require the deep anesthesia necessary for abdominal or chest surgery.

In general, for most breast surgery, the following sequence will be followed:

1. When you get to the operating room or just before you are brought there, an IV, an intravenous infusion, will be started. A needle, which is connected by tubing to a plastic container through which fluids and any intravenous anesthesia will be administered, will be placed in your arm.

2. You will be given an intravenous medication such as sodium pentothal. This drug puts you to sleep instantly, though its effects last for a relatively short time.

3. Once you are asleep, the anesthesiologist will place a mask over your nose and mouth, and administer an anesthetic gas such as nitrous oxide or ethrane. This gas will keep you asleep and also keep you from feeling any pain.

4. Anesthesia will continue to be administered as long as the surgery is in progress.

5. Throughout the surgery the anesthesiologist will be carefully monitoring your "vital signs" (heart rate, blood pressure, and respiration), making sure that your body's systems are functioning well.

THE SURGICAL PROCEDURES

MASTECTOMY

WHAT IS A MASTECTOMY?

Mastectomy is the surgical removal of the breast.

WHAT ARE THE TYPES OF MASTECTOMIES?

Modified radical, radical, total, and partial mastectomies are the general categories. As we have seen, *lumpectomy* is the term in common use when only a limited portion of the entire breast is removed. *Breast conservation* is another way of expressing it. You may hear the term *Halsted* used to describe a radical mastectomy, and *simple* used in place of *total*. The circumstances under which each type of surgery is appropriate are discussed below.

Modified Radical Mastectomy

We begin with the modified radical mastectomy because it is the mastectomy most commonly performed in the treatment of breast cancer. In fact, because it has the best long-term results with the fewest complications, it is the surgical technique against which the effectiveness of all other treatments for breast cancer are currently measured.

A "modified radical," as it is often referred to, consists of the removal of:

- The entire breast that we can actually see protruding from the chest
- The nonprotruding breast tissue that extends toward the breastbone, the collarbone, the lowest ribs, and back toward the muscle at the side of the body, the latissimus dorsi
- The lymph nodes in the armpit
- The minor pectoral muscle, removed only if it is diseased or interferes with the removal of the lymph nodes. The loss of this muscle is barely perceptible afterward. The major pec-

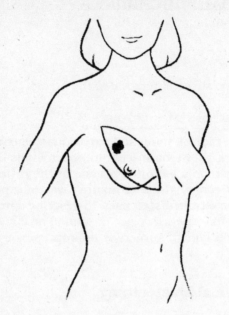

Modified radical mastectomy

toral muscle that forms the chest wall underneath the breast is not removed in a modified radical procedure. (See Radical Mastectomy, page 117.)

THE INCISION

The actual surgery should be tailored to the patient's anatomy, taking into consideration the position of the tumor and of any previous biopsy, as well as any plans for reconstruction. The incision goes from the border of the breastbone toward the armpit. It is in the shape of an ellipse—we try to avoid a vertical incision and we try to keep it slightly away from the breastbone so the scar won't be visible in low-cut clothing. Though we also hope to avoid creating any unsightly folds, unfortunately this often does occur in heavier women.

THE SURGICAL PROCEDURE

The skin and the layer of fat beneath it are cut with a scalpel or an electrocautery. A laser, a surgical instrument that uses a narrow beam of intense energy, is sometimes used for breast surgery. I don't think it has any advantages. You can achieve the same precision with a scalpel that you get with a laser, and using a laser prolongs the time the surgery takes.

The breast is then removed from the underlying muscles of the chest wall, along with the covering (fascia) that forms the "sac" that envelops the breast tissue. The major pectoral muscle is not removed.

THE AXILLARY LYMPH NODES

Why remove the nodes?

No matter where in the breast a cancer may be located, the lymphatic system of the breast drains primarily into the lymph nodes of the axilla, the armpit. For that reason it is crucial that we examine these underarm lymph nodes to see whether cancer is present. The only way to do this is to remove them, since studies have shown that one-third of the time, even the most experienced physicians aren't able to detect, simply by palpation, whether or not there is cancer in the nodes.

Lymph-node involvement is the single most important factor in planning treatment of breast cancer and in assessing prognosis. As we saw on page 40, it is vital to the process of staging, the essential measuring tool in the treatment of cancer.

Where are the lymph nodes that drain the breast?

The lymph nodes of the breast start in what is sometimes called the tail, the breast tissue that extends up toward the axilla. The nodes in this area are called **Level I** nodes. **Level II** nodes are located just beneath the pectoralis minor. **Level III** nodes are at the apex of the armpit, beyond the pectoralis minor muscle.

The nodes are not arranged in a neat trail, like pearls on a string, but are instead embedded in fat pads. And in this fact lies

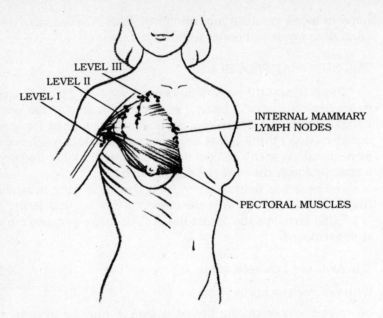

LEVEL III
LEVEL II
LEVEL I

INTERNAL MAMMARY
LYMPH NODES

PECTORAL MUSCLES

The lymphatic system of the breast

the answer to many of the questions women have about lymph-node excision. Because the nodes are embedded in fat,

- We cannot take a sample of a few specific nodes.
- We cannot predict in advance exactly how many nodes we will get.
- We cannot take the same number from all patients.
- We cannot tell accurately the total number of nodes any individual has or, therefore, the percentage that have been removed or that are cancerous.

Specific information about the nodes is not available immediately after the surgery. It is only after the pathology report that we can tell how many nodes were analyzed and how many were cancerous. In fact, this is all we need to know: the most accurate prediction of outcome arises out of the *number* of nodes involved, not the percentage.

How are the axillary nodes removed?

1. As the breast is being separated from the muscle, the axilla is approached through the same incision.

2. Fat pads, usually from Levels I and II, are removed by separating them from the adjacent structures: the vein that lies in the axilla, the nerves, and the chest wall.

3. In a modified radical, the nodes on Level III are rarely removed. If there is reason to believe they are diseased, however, we remove the pectoralis minor so that we can more easily reach these Level III nodes.

4. The pads of fat, along with the breast tissue that was removed, are sent to the pathologist for analysis.

How is the surgery completed?

1. After the breast and nodes have been removed, plastic tubes are placed beneath the skin of the breast and the pectoral muscle. These tubes are used to drain the fluid that will collect in the spaces created by the surgery. At the

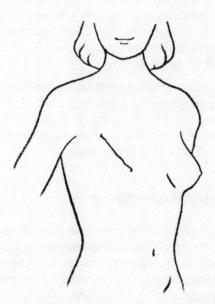

Completed modified radical mastectomy

places where the tubes emerge, they are sutured to the skin and attached to a small bulblike device in which there is a vacuum that fills with this fluid.

2. The incision is closed with absorbable sutures or with metal staples. Though there are varying degrees of skill among surgeons, the aim is to close an incision so that when it heals, the scar will be thin and flat on the chest wall. The incision for a modified radical may be fairly long, depending on breast size, and it may be under tension, depending on its placement on the chest. Therefore, the wound may not heal absolutely uniformly. Still, it is important to remember that there are surgeons whose results, from an aesthetic point of view, are regularly quite good.

     All mastectomies should be planned with breast reconstruction in mind, whether or not specific plans have been made for it at this point. It is not necessary for a plastic surgeon to be present merely for the closing of the incision. If, however, you and your surgeon have decided that you will have breast reconstruction at the same time as your mastectomy, then, of course, the plastic surgeon will be standing by. For further information on how such a decision is made and on the details of breast reconstruction, see Chapter Eleven.

3. The wound is dressed with protective bandages. I prefer to use a light dressing. I don't think you need a lot of pressure from a bulky dressing to "bind" the wound because the use of suction drains makes it possible for the skin to "stick down" to the chest wall.

Total (Simple) Mastectomy

The total (or simple) mastectomy is a procedure that is like the first part of a modified radical mastectomy. However, only the breast is removed—*not* the axillary lymph nodes. Total mastectomy is now being used with increasing frequency for *in situ* intraductal cancer.

Radical Mastectomy

The radical mastectomy involves the removal of the breast, the muscles of the chest wall, and, sometimes, so much skin that skin grafting may be necessary. This deforming breast surgery, which women feared for so many years, is rarely performed today, because most breast cancers are found early, before they have invaded the muscle. The physical and psychological results of this operation were traumatic, and very different from what we commonly achieve today.

This procedure was developed in the late nineteenth century by William S. Halsted and you may hear his name used to describe a radical mastectomy. It was the only breast surgery available until the development and use of the "modified radical" in 1948 in England, and in the 1970s in America.

Because the major pectoral muscle is removed, the natural contour of the chest wall is lost, arm mobility may be affected for a time, and breast reconstruction (see Chapter Eleven) is more difficult.

An enlarged version of this procedure removed the lymph nodes behind the breastbone as well as a segment of the ribs. Called an extended radical mastectomy, or a super-radical, it is no longer in use.

Partial Mastectomy

A partial mastectomy is the removal of part of the breast. Depending on the extent of the procedure, this may also be called wide excision or quadrantectomy. The more general and more commonly used term for preserving the breast, treating it without removing it, is *lumpectomy*. In these procedures, the cancerous tissue plus a margin of healthy tissue is removed, as are some axillary lymph nodes. The surgery is always followed by radiation treatment of the breast; and as with a mastectomy, adjuvant hormone or chemotherapy is usually used.

Breast conservation is a relatively new procedure and the surgical techniques are still developing. There may be differences in how equally competent surgeons approach these operations. The material that follows in this chapter is, of course, a description of the techniques and practices that I use. If it differs from what your surgeon plans for you, discuss that with him. His ideas may be absolutely right for you, your cancer, and your anatomy.

WIDE EXCISION

If the tumor is small in relation to the whole breast, its removal, plus the removal of about two centimeters (three-fourths of an inch) of healthy tissue all around, is called a wide excision. Sometimes, enough tissue has been taken at the time of the biopsy so that this procedure is not necessary.

QUADRANTECTOMY

If twenty to twenty-five percent of the breast (a quarter, or quadrant) is removed, along with the overlying skin, the procedure is called a quadrantectomy. Obviously, the breast will be smaller after this procedure.

WHEN DO PARTIAL MASTECTOMIES YIELD GOOD COSMETIC RESULTS?

The purpose of partial mastectomy is to cure the disease and preserve the breast. While it is safe, in many cases, to use this procedure in tumors up to four centimeters (one and a half inches) in size, other factors must also be considered:

- Removing a large tumor from a large breast may result in a nearly normal-looking breast. Taking that same size tumor out of a small breast would not yield an attractive result.
- Because we must always have a clear margin of healthy tissue, wide excisions of tumors in the center of the breast or in the areola may not yield good aesthetic results. Such tumors are better treated with mastectomy.
- If more than one tumor is present, several wide excisions may also preclude a satisfactory appearance.

SURGICAL PROCEDURE FOR PARTIAL MASTECTOMY

1. The incision for partial mastectomy must be carefully individualized to the woman's anatomy and to the size and

118

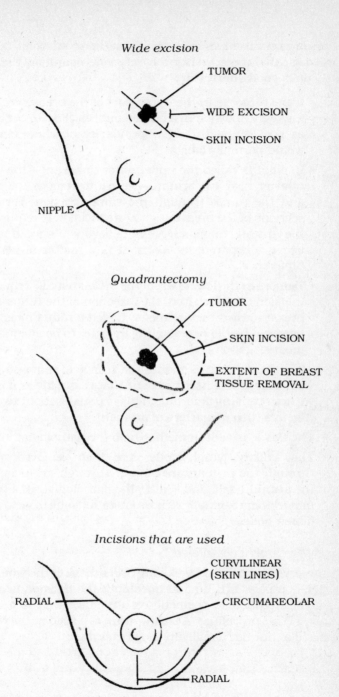

Wide excision

TUMOR

WIDE EXCISION

SKIN INCISION

NIPPLE

Quadrantectomy

TUMOR

SKIN INCISION

EXTENT OF BREAST
TISSUE REMOVAL

Incisions that are used

CURVILINEAR
(SKIN LINES)

RADIAL

CIRCUMAREOLAR

RADIAL

location of the tumor. An experienced surgeon can, in most instances, perform a very safe operation that also looks good afterward.

- If the tumor is in the upper part of the breast, we try to make the incision in a curved line, as close to the areola as possible, within the boundaries of where clothing would normally fall.

- In what is called the upper outer quadrant—the upper quarter near the armpit—we try to remove the nodes and the tumor through the same incision. For other sections of the breast, a separate incision is required for the armpit. Some surgeons believe you should always use two separate incisions. It is a matter of personal preference.

- Tumors in the lower part of the breast usually require an incision that goes from the direction of the center of the breast toward the perimeter. Called a radial incision, it need not be big or unsightly in order to be adequate for most situations.

2. After the incision is made, the tumor is removed along with a margin of healthy tissue that is as wide as possible without causing deformity. This is usually about two centimeters (three-quarters of an inch).

3. The tissue is sent immediately to the pathologist.

4. The axillary lymph nodes are then removed, either through the primary incision or through an incision in the armpit itself, and sent to the pathologist. In a partial mastectomy, I usually remove enough tissue to yield ten to fifteen nodes.

How is the surgery completed?

The surgery is completed by closing and dressing the wound as described on page 116. In a lumpectomy, the incision is closed with great attention to cosmetic results since that is a major objective of this procedure. A plastic drain is placed in the wound in the axilla, but not usually in the breast itself.

AFTER THE SURGERY

The Recovery Room

When you awaken after the surgery, you will find yourself in the recovery room with other postoperative patients.

Your condition will be carefully watched by the specialized nurses who staff these rooms. Your heart rate, blood pressure, and respiration will be monitored, and you will be kept in this room until you are fully awake and your condition has stabilized.

If you feel any pain, tell the recovery room nurse. Orders for pain medication will have been written by the surgeon or the anesthesiologist, and the nurse will be ready to give the drug to you if you need it.

You may feel cold after you awaken from the surgery. Shivering is part of the recovery process after anesthesia. Ask for more blankets if you need them. You may want to bring a warm blanket with you to the hospital, in case there is not an ample supply. I advise my patients to do this, though you will not be permitted to use it in the recovery room.

How Long Is the Hospital Stay?

Because of government and hospital reimbursement regulations, the current trend is to keep patients in the hospital for as short a time as is feasible. In fact, many patients welcome the opportunity to go home earlier thanks to improvements in anesthesia and pain medications. Nowadays that means the following:

- For modified radical mastectomy, usually about three days.
- For modified radicals with reconstruction, usually three to six days, depending on the method used.
- For partial mastectomy or lumpectomy with axillary dissection, usually overnight. In some parts of the country these have become same-day ambulatory surgery procedures.

Removing Drains, Sutures, and Staples

- After a modified radical mastectomy, we usually remove one of the drains on the second or third day after surgery and leave the other drain in place until after the patient goes

121

home from the hospital. It is removed during a subsequent office visit, when the wound is no longer draining. A drain may be needed for one to two weeks. Do not worry if it needs to remain longer; this does not mean that anything is wrong. After the drains are removed, if fluid collects at the site of surgery it can be easily removed, with minimal discomfort, in the doctor's office, using a syringe and needle.

Where the breast has been conserved, drains are ordinarily used only in the armpit and are removed either before discharge from the hospital or during a subsequent office visit, after the wound has stopped draining.

- Because we ordinarily use sutures that are absorbed into the body, there is no need to remove them.
- Staples are removed at the time of an office visit.

Pain

Aside from some pain that may occur from an incision in the armpit, neither partial nor modified radical mastectomies cause much discomfort. Because this is a major concern, I have talked about it with literally thousands of women and have asked them to describe to me what these procedures feel like. Almost every woman reports "an uncomfortable day of surgery and first night, but no real pain," and my patients seem to use very little medication after that first night.

Though it is not pain, many women feel a sensation of tightness at the site of the surgery after a modified radical mastectomy. This feeling markedly improves after the first few weeks, though some feeling of tightness may linger for several months.

Numbness

During the removal of the lymph nodes, we come in contact with the nerves that control sensation at the back of the underarm area. You may, therefore, experience temporary or permanent numbness at this site.

With a modified radical mastectomy, there is a general numbness of the chest wall within the area of incision. Most women say that the numbness improves in a few months and eventually disappears.

Infection

Since women know that the lymph nodes are part of the immune system, they quite understandably worry that the removal of underarm nodes will increase their risk of infection. The truth of the matter is that there are many groups of lymph nodes throughout the body and, proportionately, the number that is taken during an axillary dissection is insignificant.

Though there is no general impairment of the immunological system, axillary excision does interfere with the lymphatic drainage of the arm. Because the arm is now less able to handle infection,

- Avoid going to manicurists.
- Don't cut or push at the cuticles of your own fingernails. This is the place where most arm infections start.
- If blood samples have to be taken in future examinations, ask that the doctor or technician use the arm whose lymph nodes are intact. Though it is unlikely that this procedure will cause infection, there is no inconvenience in using the other arm for this purpose.

Many physicians say you should avoid allowing your blood pressure to be measured on the affected arm, but there is no evidence that this causes any trouble.

The fact is that infections develop only rarely, though any needle puncture or breaking of the skin can cause problems. In addition to manicure incidents, the most common offenders are burns, thorns, embedded particles of steel wool, and insect bites.

If, by any chance, you notice any of the following symptoms, call the surgeon. He will prescribe antibiotics that will usually clear up any infection quickly and safely.

- Splotchy redness on the arm or chest
- Pain or tenderness, often starting along the inner side of the elbow but at times severe throughout the arm
- Pain at the front of the chest wall

KVCC KALAMAZOO VALLEY COMMUNITY COLLEGE LIBRARY

Edema

Swelling, or edema, of the arm used to be more common when radical mastectomy was followed by radiation therapy. This combination often interfered with lymph drainage in the arm. With the modified radical mastectomy, however, more lymphatic channels are left intact. Only about five percent of women who have had this surgery develop troublesome problems with edema. With lumpectomies, such edema is even less frequent. You should call your surgeon if it develops.

Phlebitis

Following an incision in the axilla or the chest, even that of a breast biopsy, a very superficial vein of the affected arm may sometimes develop a clot. Called phlebothrombosis, this condition is not serious because it is not in a vital part of the vascular system.

When this type of phlebitis is present, you may find that after you have already recovered the full range of motion of your arm (see below), you are suddenly able to do less. You may feel as if there is a wire in your arm that is keeping you from fully extending it. Though these symptoms can seem alarming, treatment is not usually required. The condition can be uncomfortable, however, and can take four to six weeks to disappear.

Activity

It seems to me that women recover most quickly and best if they begin exercising as soon as possible after the surgery. Patients sometimes worry that the stitches won't hold, or that the wound will open, or that some other mishap will occur.

As a rule, mastectomy incisions on the chest do not pull apart. You have to be more selective in the kinds of exercises you do if there was an axillary incision. (No one would want to lift weights or serve overhand in tennis, for example, with an unhealed wound under the arm.) If you have any questions about a particular activity, discuss it with the surgeon.

What follows is not an inflexible schedule, but one that reflects the pace and level of activity under which patients seem to do best. It may be slightly altered if there is breast reconstruction at the same time as the surgery:

- Get out of bed within a few hours after the surgery.
- Begin arm exercises (see below) the morning after surgery.
- Resume a normal schedule of activity a few days after lumpectomy.
- Resume a normal schedule of activity two to three weeks after mastectomy.

ARM EXERCISES

Nowadays, most women do not find that the range of motion of their arm is limited after breast surgery. Therefore, exercise specifically for arm strengthening is not necessary.

All we do in my practice is to ask women to do simple stretches, while seated, starting the morning after surgery. You should be able to do them fairly easily within a few days. In the first exercise, grasp both hands together in your lap, lift your arms—elbows out—over your head, and finally rest your clasped hands at the back of your neck. In the next exercise, as in calisthenics or aerobics, bring the arms up, out, forward, and down. First raise them straight up, then extend them horizontally, bring them forward and together directly in front of you, and finally lower them onto your lap.

WHEN CAN I BATHE?

You can take a shower when the drains and the staples or any sutures have been removed. You can take a bath when the wound has healed, or earlier, if a waterproof dressing is used.

REACH TO RECOVERY

The American Cancer Society trains women who have themselves had breast cancer to act as volunteers in helping current patients. It can be very reassuring to talk to someone who has "been there" and also to receive printed information on matters like the use of prostheses (see pages 193–194) and other postoperative questions you may have. Someone in your surgeon's office can usually put you in touch with the Reach to Recovery organization if you think it would be helpful.

HOW DO I KNOW WHICH TYPE OF SURGERY IS RIGHT FOR ME?

Our basic job is to get rid of the cancer and prevent its spread and recurrence, if possible while preserving the breast. In order to accomplish that task, we have to understand the nature or pathology of the malignancy; its stage, including its size and how much it has spread; its location in the breast; and the size of the breast itself. We also have to give serious consideration to what you yourself prefer.

The following sections describe the general circumstances under which each type of surgery is appropriate.

Stage 0 Cancer

Stage 0 cancers are noninfiltrating cancers confined to the lobules and ducts.

- Lobular carcinoma *in situ* (LCIS), generally speaking, requires no surgery after the biopsy. It should, however, be very carefully watched. Mammography and a physical examination by a doctor should be regularly scheduled because this *in situ* cancer is what we call a marker of great risk. Twenty percent of women with this symptom develop infiltrating cancers over a twenty-year period and there is a likelihood that both breasts are at risk.

- In the past, duct cell carcinoma *in situ* (DCIS) was usually discovered after a biopsy for a nipple discharge or ulceration. With the recent improvements in mammography, we are able to pick up very early abnormalities, and now over twenty percent of the women we treat for breast cancer have DCIS.

To treat DCIS, we do a total mastectomy (without lymph node removal) or we do a lumpectomy followed by radiation therapy. Which procedure to choose poses a dilemma. We know that if we treat DCIS with mastectomy, we can achieve close to one hundred percent success. If we preserve the breast with a wide excision and radiotherapy, there is a one-percent-a-year recurrence rate. Of those women who have a recurrence, half can be successfully treated with mastectomy. The other half will have infil-trating disease. Some of them will be cured, but some lives will be lost.

Many women and their doctors say, "If there is any risk of recurrence at all, do a mastectomy." Others decide that one per-cent a year is an acceptable risk. They are opting for as wide an excision as can be done to avoid deformity, along with radiation therapy.

As we will see below, invasive cancers are treated with lump-ectomy, node removal, and radiation. It seems paradoxical that cases of DCIS—that is, of noninvasive cancer—are often treated with mastectomy because of the one hundred percent cure rate. As one of my patients said, "Is the loss of my breast the reward I get for finding cancer before it has spread?"

There are studies now under way to try to resolve this dichot-omy, and to find out whether, in some cases of DCIS, wide exci-sion alone is adequate treatment. In the meantime, if you have an *in situ* ductal cancer, you and your doctor will have to carefully discuss and weigh your treatment options. We are not yet at the point where, as in early lobular cancers, we can monitor and observe and, at least, delay surgery. But treatment for intraductal carcinomas *in situ* can and should be individualized and the options carefully weighed as to their physical and emotional consequences.

Stage I and Stage II Cancers

The discussion of treatment for these cancers is best begun with a quote from "the horse's mouth," a conference convened by the National Institutes of Health (NIH) to evaluate available scientific information and to "resolve safety and efficacy issues related to biomedical technology." According to the findings of this NIH Consensus Conference on early, invasive breast cancer, in June 1990, "Breast conservation treatment is an appropriate method of primary therapy for the majority of women with Stages I and II breast cancer and is preferable because it provides survival rates equivalent to those of total mastectomy [modified radical] and axillary dissection while preserving the breast."

To clarify, lumpectomy with axillary dissection and radiation therapy is the preferable treatment for small infiltrating cancers of either the lobules or the ducts.

There are, however, circumstances where mastectomy is the treatment advised for Stage I and Stage II cancers:

- More than one cancerous tumor in the breast
- Multiple areas of microcalcification (see page 77) in the breast
- A relatively large tumor in a small breast or a tumor in or near the center of the breast
- Considerable axillary lymph-node involvement

In addition, some physicians consider mastectomy the preferred treatment in the following circumstances:

- Extensive intraductal cancer *in situ* within and adjacent to the primary tumor
- An infiltrating cancer plus a considerable amount of intraductal cancer

Under certain circumstances, we may recommend a bilateral mastectomy when there is lobular cancer *in situ*:

- If there have been recurrent lumps that required biopsy
- If mammograms show calcifications that are difficult to interpret
- If there is an extremely strong family history of breast cancer

Stage III Cancers

We have, up until now, been discussing early, relatively small cancers. As we saw in Chapter Three, some women come for treatment with more advanced disease. In such cases, the cancer may be in the skin of the breast, it may be of the inflammatory type, it may be accompanied by extensive lymph-node involvement, or the tumor may be over five centimeters (about two inches) in size.

For Stage III cancers, chemotherapy (see Chapter Ten) is the first treatment. It is used to treat inflammatory cancer and also to shrink a large tumor to operable size. Surgery, usually a modified radical mastectomy, is performed after the tumor has shrunk.

Stage IV Cancers

Stage IV cancers have spread beyond the breast and the axillary lymph nodes to other places in the body. They are treated primarily with chemotherapy. Surgery—lumpectomy or modified radical mastectomy—or radiation therapy may sometimes be used to assist in local tumor control.

It is important to say here that I have patients in my practice who came to me with a large tumor and who have done well, usually with chemotherapy followed by surgery. In a few instances, where the tumor was inoperable, some women have survived for many years on long-term chemotherapy.

Cancer in Pregnancy

As we saw in Chapter Three, breast cancer in pregnant women tends to be discovered at a later stage than cancer in other women. Our general approach is to "abort the cancer, not the baby." However, when cancer is discovered during the first trimester, women usually choose to terminate the pregnancy and then to promptly seek the most appropriate treatment for the disease.

During the second trimester or later, a mastectomy can be safely performed. We do not use radiation with pregnant women so as not to risk the well-being of the fetus. Chemotherapy may be started only in the very last weeks of pregnancy.

Treatment Options

To summarize the sequence of treatment that may be recommended for all stages of breast cancer:

TREATMENT

STAGE 0

LOBULAR CARCINOMA *IN SITU*

1. Biopsy
2. Observation
3. Possible hormone therapy (see page 250)

or

1. Bilateral mastectomy
2. Breast reconstruction

DUCTAL CARCINOMA *IN SITU*

1. Biopsy
2. Mastectomy

or

1. Wide excision with observation only (experimental)

or

1. Wide excision plus radiation

STAGE I

1. Biopsy
2. Partial (lumpectomy) or modified radical mastectomy
3. Axillary dissection
4. If mastectomy, possible breast reconstruction
5. If lumpectomy, radiation therapy
6. Possible hormone therapy or chemotherapy

STAGE II

1. Biopsy
2. Lumpectomy or modified radical mastectomy
3. Axillary dissection
4. If mastectomy, possible breast reconstruction
5. If lumpectomy, radiation therapy
6. Hormone therapy or chemotherapy

STAGE III

1. Biopsy
2. Course of chemotherapy
3. Modified radical mastectomy
4. Continued chemotherapy
5. Radiation therapy

STAGE IV

1. Biopsy
2. Course of chemotherapy
3. If appropriate, lumpectomy
   or
   Modified radical mastectomy
4. Continued chemotherapy

CHAPTER

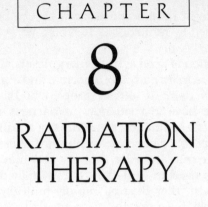

8

RADIATION THERAPY

❧◊❧

To destroy cancer cells, radiation therapy most commonly uses electromagnetic radiation, consisting of X rays and gamma rays. It also uses what is called particulate radiation, waves of electronic particles such as electrons, neutrons, and protons.

What is electromagnetic radiation? Waves of energy from various sources, electromagnetic rays include ordinary light, X rays, and gamma rays. The rays used in therapy have special properties:

Though sunlight can shine through a fairly sheer window curtain, X rays and gamma rays actually have the ability to penetrate solids. It is this property that allows us to use them to treat tissue within the body and to "see through" the skin to what is inside. The dentist, for example, uses minute levels of radiation to examine our teeth. In fact, he uses a lot less than one rad, the unit of measure of radiation absorbed by the body. About the same level is used by radiologists to whom we go for other diagnostic X rays.

When radiation is used at high energy levels, it has the ability to destroy what is in its path, both normal and abnormal tissues. Why then are we using it to treat people who have had cancer?

Because we have learned how to harness this enormous power in the battle against cancer. Think of a radiation device as a high-tech, superbly focused searchlight that can be accurately aimed at cancer cells in order that its rays may destroy them. While the doses used in radiation therapy may damage normal cells in their path, they *destroy* rapidly multiplying malignant cells. Normal cells have the ability to repair themselves, and in the treatment of breast cancer, the side effects are local—limited to the specific area of the radiation and not involving the rest of the body.

THE COURSE OF RADIATION THERAPY

After Lumpectomy

Women who have had lumpectomies, almost without exception, are now treated with radiation. That statement inevitably raises two good questions:

1. If the cancer was removed, why do I need further treatment?

The decision to use radiation is based on overwhelming evidence that there is an unacceptably high rate of recurrence in the affected breast when the cancer is treated by lumpectomy alone. This rate can be reduced three- to four-fold when we add radiation therapy. In fact, by combining lumpectomy and radiation, we can get results that are comparable to those from mastectomy—while still preserving the breast.

2. If radiation therapy is so effective, why did I need the surgery in the first place?

The smaller the malignancy, the better radiation works. By surgically removing all the cancer we can detect, the radiation is left to deal primarily with undetected microscopic disease. That is why, in doing lumpectomies, we perform the widest excisions possible, with clear margins all around.

In addition, by surgically removing all the cancer we can find, we make it possible to use doses of radiation that are small enough to do only minimal damage to normal tissue.

After Mastectomy

Though radiation is not commonly used with mastectomy, sometimes when a tumor is large, or when the surgeon has not been able to get a wide enough margin around it, radiation will be used to make sure all the disease is eradicated.

Lymph-Node Treatment

Radiation may be used to treat the lymph nodes behind the breastbone or above the collarbone if those nodes are at high risk of containing cancer cells. For example, we would suspect this to be the case if a great deal of cancer is found at the inner side of the breast or in the axilla.

Extremely Large Tumors

When the tumor is too large to be operated on, chemotherapy is commonly used to shrink it to operable size. Then, following surgery, because of the relatively high risk of recurrence at this stage of the disease, radiation may be employed to attack any microscopic malignancy that may have escaped surgical removal. If a large tumor does not shrink to operable size after chemotherapy, radiation may also be used; but after surgery in these cases, no additional radiation is employed.

Local Recurrence

Occasionally, after a mastectomy, a small malignancy may appear at the site of the original disease, or in the skin or on the underlying muscle of the chest wall. Because there is no apparent

135

spread to other parts of the body, this is called a local recurrence. The tumor is removed, and radiation is used to sterilize a wider area of the chest wall. Chemotherapy and/or hormone therapy may be given before or after the radiation.

Metastasis

When breast cancer has spread to other parts of the body, chemotherapy is both the first line of defense against further progression and the front-line attack against the existing disease (see Chapter Ten). Sometimes, however, cancer that has spread to the bones may cause pain and bone destruction. Radiation therapy of the affected bone is very successful in relieving this condition.

WHO IS THE RIGHT PHYSICIAN?

You must go to a *radiotherapist*, or *radiation oncologist*, a physician trained in the planning and administration of radiation for medical treatment. There are radiation therapists whose particular area of interest and expertise is the treatment of breast cancer. This is the kind of person you are looking for.

She should have had training and experience in radiation therapy and be either board-certified or board-eligible. Board-certified physicians have passed an examination in radiation therapy. Board-eligible physicians have had the training and experience, but have not taken the examination.

Finding a qualified radiotherapist, however, is only part of the job. The treatment facility must have available to it the services of a qualified *radiation physicist* who has a Ph.D. or M.S. degree. Such a person is key to the precise planning of the radiation therapy.

There must also be licensed *radiation technologists* at the facility who are qualified to operate the radiation therapy equipment.

There should also be trained *radiation therapy nurses*, who work closely with the physicians and the technologists, and who are knowledgeable about the treatment and able to answer many of the questions you may have. Since you will be seeing the technologist and the nurse every day for a considerable period of time, you should feel comfortable with their manner and behavior as well as with their competence.

How do you know the radiation facility is staffed with competent personnel? All states require that radiation departments or facilities have qualified physicians and other technical personnel. The credentials of these individuals are routinely reviewed at regular intervals by local and state agencies. The certificates of education and certification of each of the staff members should be conspicuously posted in the office. If you do not see every certification you're looking for, ask. It's worth any momentary embarrassment to make sure you are at the right place for your treatment.

WHERE DO YOU FIND THE RADIOTHERAPIST?

Radiotherapists and other radiation specialists are found in hospital or cancer-center radiotherapy departments and also in private practice. Because extremely fine skills are required to destroy the cancer yet avoid damaging the body, finding a good radiotherapist takes very careful consideration. It is so important that it may be worth making arrangements to receive the treatments in another community if there is not an excellent facility near where you live.

As you will see, treatment lasts for several weeks, so this may not be a suggestion that is easy to follow; but the effort may be worth it in terms of the quality of treatment, the results, and the follow-up. In fact, when we first started doing lumpectomies several years ago, relatively few radiotherapists were experienced with this new way of treating breast cancer, so it was quite common for women to go to another city for the weeks of their treatment. Even today, when there is no excellent local facility, some women spend Monday through Friday in the city where the radiotherapy facility is located and then go home for the weekend.

Your surgeon will usually refer you to a radiotherapist to whom he has already sent patients and whose work he respects. Even so, carefully consider whether this is the right doctor and the right facility for you. Refer again to Chapter Two and review the material on finding and evaluating a doctor. If you have any questions about the radiotherapist, by all means discuss them with your surgeon before you go for treatment.

INFORMED CONSENT

At the beginning of your first visit, you will be asked to sign an informed-consent form that will specify the type of treatment you will be receiving and the possible risks and side effects. It will ask you to certify that the procedure and its risks have been explained to you and that you agree to the treatment.

Read the form carefully. If there is any discrepancy between what you have been told your treatment will be and what is stated on the form, ask that the language be explained to you clearly enough so that you understand it or, if necessary, ask that it be changed. You should feel comfortable about the form and not have to worry about any fine print.

However, as we saw when we looked at informed consent in the chapter on surgery, though the form plays some role in protecting the physician from later charges of malpractice, and though it spells out for the patient the precise nature of the treatment, in the end, regardless of what the form says, doctors, like other professionals, are responsible for their work.

EQUIPMENT

A machine called a linear accelerator, which employs electrical current to generate X rays and electrons, is now commonly used to deliver radiation therapy.

Also in use is a cobalt machine, which emits gamma rays from a radioactive source of the element cobalt.

Generally speaking, either device may be used to treat breast cancer. The linear accelerator is capable of producing more powerful X rays and may be used for the "boost" treatment, at the site of the tumor, that is discussed below.

THE TREATMENT

Planning

Though the radiotherapist may be consulted before the tumor is even removed, you certainly will be seeing her about two weeks after your surgery. Your surgeon should have thoroughly discussed your case with the radiotherapist by the time of your first visit. He will have sent her copies of your preoperative mammogram, the results of any tests you may have had, and the pathology report. (In addition, some radiotherapists prefer to review the pathology slides themselves.) The surgeon should also have told the radiotherapist any pertinent details of your medical history or of the operation.

How do you know that this exchange of information has taken place before you get to the radiation facility? Ask. If the surgeon has already done this groundwork, if the radiotherapist is well prepared to receive you, nothing has been lost by your question. If not, you will perhaps have nudged the process along.

Pinpointing the Area

Your first visit to the radiotherapist will take about an hour and will be devoted to accurately determining the area to be treated. This planning requires the use of specially designed equipment, as well as computer technology, to precisely locate and mark the parts of the body that are to receive radiation—the fields—and to determine the angles at which the radiation will be delivered.

A wire model of the breast contour is constructed and then transferred to graph paper to outline the volume to be treated.

This region on your chest is marked with water-soluble ink, and a treatment simulator is then used as a stand-in for the actual treatment machine.

Think again of the searchlight and the circle of light it casts. The radiation source also emits its rays in a particular shape and depth—*in its own geometry* is the term often used. A simulator, also referred to as a localizer simulator, is used to duplicate precisely where the radiation will go in your body. How will the machine be angled for treatment? What will be the port of entry of the radiation? The size of the port? In relation to the radiation's range, where are the vital organs? The lungs? The heart? Using a simulator before taking X-ray pictures is like a dress rehearsal before the actual performance.

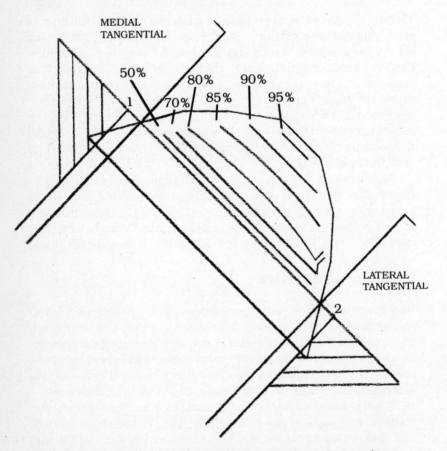

Computer-generated treatment plan showing the radiation dose distribution (in percentages) within the breast. This will be used for prescribing the amount of radiation to be given.

In addition to the simulator, a CAT scan (see page 69) may be employed if the size of the breast or the position of the tumor makes it difficult to get the necessary detailed information.

The radiation physicist then feeds the information into a computer that has been programmed to calculate the distribution of the radiation in the volume to be treated. This helps determine the proper field size, and the angles at which the radiation should be delivered to achieve the most exposure to the breast and the least exposure to other tissue. This process of localizing the radiation area is carried out meticulously to assure that we destroy any cancer cells without exposing the heart, lungs, or ribs to unnecessary radiation.

Marking

Once this work has been accomplished, the radiation therapist will mark the area of treatment on your skin with lines of indelible ink or, more commonly, with tiny tattoo marks no bigger than the head of a pin. These marks enable the therapist to reproduce the daily treatment in precisely the same area.

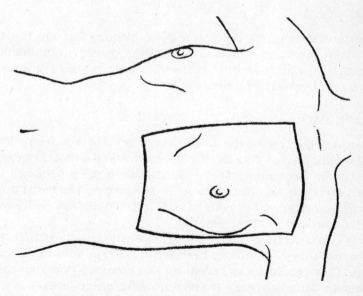

Marking or tattooing the area to be irradiated

141

The tattooing may prick a bit, but it does not really cause much discomfort. Usually, the dots are minute, and because tattooing cannot wash off, you don't have to worry about bathing.

Some women do seem to hate the idea that the site of their cancer will be forever marked on their skin, although lasers can now be used to remove the tattoos. If you feel that way, ask that ink be used. However, "indelible" ink does eventually wash away. You need to avoid washing the area too vigorously, and you have to make sure that when the marking is done initially or freshened up later, it doesn't get on your clothes.

Schedule

For the first weeks of your treatment, Phase One, the entire breast is treated, the whole area that would ordinarily be encompassed by a mastectomy. Generally speaking, the underarm area does not have to be treated.

In a second phase, most women will get a supplemental treatment, called a boost, that concentrates the radiation in the area where the tumor was located.

PHASE ONE

Treatments are given five days a week, Monday through Friday, for about five to six weeks. The weekend pause is not only for reasons of convenience but because normal cells need a little time to recover between treatments.

PHASE TWO

Immediately following the first course of radiotherapy, the patient will receive a boost dose in that area of the breast that contained the tumor. Depending on the planned dose, treatment will be given every day for one to two-and-a-half weeks. The boost dose is now commonly administered by external radiation, by X rays, gamma rays, or electron beam.

It can also be given in the form of internal radiation, by inserting tubes containing radioactive material into the tumor area. This procedure is becoming less common now that surgeons are removing more tissue during lumpectomies.

142

Inserting the tubes is a surgical procedure that can be performed by the radiotherapist alone or in association with the surgeon. It requires local or general anesthesia. The tubes must remain in the breast for two or three days, during which time the radioactive material emits the desired amount of radiation. The patient is hospitalized; and nurses, doctors, and visitors are at some risk of radiation exposure and cannot be in close contact with you for an extended period of time. A lead shield is placed between the patient and visitors to lessen exposure; adult visitors can safely stay behind the shield for thirty to forty minutes.

Keeping Your Appointments

It is important that you go for all your scheduled treatments. You would not take one antibiotic pill if you had a strep throat and think you had been cured. To make sure all the cancer cells have been destroyed, the full course of treatment is necessary. If you or the doctor must miss a day, you will be asked to make it up so that you get the entire planned dose.

It is this aspect of radiation therapy that women find most troublesome. They often ask why the full course of radiotherapy cannot be given in one or two treatments.

Though having to go to the radiotherapist's facility every day, as if you were going to a job, can seem daunting, the treatments must be spread over several weeks so that the daily radiation dose is relatively small. In this way, the total dose can be achieved with less damage to the skin and other tissues than a single high dose might produce.

How Much Radiation Will I Receive?

The total dose will be calculated at the time of your first planning visit. Questions like these will be considered by the radiotherapist and the radiation physicist:

- What is the total dose the entire breast should receive?
- What dose should be given in the boost?

143

- For how many weeks is it estimated that treatment will continue?
- For how many minutes will each treatment be administered?

Also taken into consideration are the size of the breast, the location and size of the tumor, the involvement of the lymph nodes, and the stage of the disease. In general, during the first phase of treatment, a total of 4,600 to 5,000 rads is given to the whole breast over a period of five to six weeks. The boost dose is usually 1,600 to 2,000 rads, given over about two to three weeks.

A Companion

Take someone, preferably your personal advocate, with you to the first, planning visit, as well as to your first treatment. As in other aspects of your treatment, such a person can give you moral support, can help you ask questions, and also may help you remember the information you will receive. These treatments are painless and are not associated with uncomfortable side effects, so you will probably find that you won't need anyone with you after the first couple of times.

What Is the Daily Routine?

1. You will be given a clean paper or cloth gown and asked to remove all clothing and jewelry from the upper part of your body.

2. You will be taken to the treatment room and will be asked to lie down on the table beneath the machine with your arm raised and supported with an armrest. Usually you will be flat on your back, though sometimes you may be asked to lie on your side.

3. Once the technologist and radiotherapist have positioned you for the first field to be treated and adjusted the angle of the machine, they will leave the room, closing the door behind them. The machine will be turned on and you will be asked to lie completely still, though, unlike the routine

during X-ray pictures, you can breathe normally during your treatment, which can take a minute or two.

Do not worry about being left alone. You are being monitored by closed-circuit television and there is a microphone in the room so that you can be heard outside if you have something to say.

4. After the first radiation has been administered, the technologist will return and position you for the next field of treatment. Usually one or two fields are irradiated each day.

5. The whole process takes about twenty minutes, though the radiation treatment itself takes only a fraction of that time.

6. At the time of the first treatment, and then at intervals during the course of your treatment, a blood test will be taken to make sure that the radiation is not affecting your blood count—something that rarely happens with breast radiation.

7. You will be asked to avoid using deodorants, powder, or perfumes, because some of their ingredients may cause skin irritation during treatment. If you have not had a tattoo, you will also be cautioned to only lightly wash the area where your body has been marked to avoid rubbing off the ink. You may resume normal activities after treatment is completed.

Will It Hurt?

Radiation treatment does not seem to cause anyone any pain. A few women say that they feel some tingling or warmth in the area being treated but even that sensation seems to be rare.

Will I Be Sick During the Course of Treatment?

You can carry on your normal life to a great extent while you are receiving radiation therapy. There are rarely any really troublesome problems, and only a few discomforts:

- Think of radiation as giving you a sunburn, not just of the skin, but of the entire area the treatment encompasses. As the tissues absorb the radiation, they tend to retain water, so, as in a sunburn, there may be some swelling. For that reason, you may want to wear a cotton T-shirt rather than a bra or under a bra during the weeks you are being treated.

- In addition to the swelling, your skin may get a little red—again, as if you had a sunburn. This is particularly likely to happen after the fourth or fifth week of treatment.

- There is some pattern of increasing fatigue as the treatments continue. Part of this may be due to the strain of getting to the radiation facility every day, but it is so prevalent that there is reason to believe it is also related to the generalized effect of the treatment, particularly if more areas than the breast alone are being irradiated. Try to go with what your body is telling you. Don't radically change your life, but, especially toward the end of your treatment, program yourself to allow time to rest when you need to.

What Are the Long-Term Side Effects?

The question that causes the most concern is, Will the radiation treatment itself cause a later cancer? There is no evidence that it does, either at the site of the treatment or in the other breast.

In the past, when low-energy X rays were used, there was some increased incidence of a disease called sarcoma, a malignancy of blood vessels, bones, or connective tissues. With modern radiation equipment that produces high-energy X rays, these cancers are almost unheard-of.

Younger women, in particular, worry about the effects of this therapy on their reproductive system. It has been estimated that during the course of treatment, the ovaries do receive from thirty to forty rads of radiation, depending on the patient's size and the site of the treatment. This is due to scattered radiation within the body, and it cannot be decreased by adding lead protection. Thirty to forty rads are not considered biologically significant. Neither menstrual periods nor fertility is affected.

You will probably not be able to nurse a baby with a breast that has received radiation. The other breast will be able to lactate, and some women who have had this treatment have nursed their babies.

Very occasionally, radiation can cause a hairline fracture of a rib. This doesn't usually cause problems, and there may be no evidence of its presence until it shows up on an X ray. Similarly, radiation can sometimes injure the lungs. *Properly planned and administered radiation therapy rarely causes these problems.*

Most swelling of the breast usually disappears after a few weeks, but if the boost radiation was near the nipple and areola, the swelling may take a longer time to subside. The skin in these areas is much thinner and therefore harder to repair. Also, if a tumor near the center of the breast was removed, there is a greater likelihood of long-term edema from damaged lymphatics.

Some women report a feeling of warmth that continues for several months after the treatment.

You may find some changes in sensation, but there is no uniformity to this reaction; some women say their breast is much more sensitive, others say it is less so.

There are some cosmetic side effects, but these are usually quite minor: the superficial layers of skin will die and this will leave a slight discoloration; the skin may darken and thicken slightly. Use a vitamin A and D cream or other non-irritating preparation to moisturize the skin. Don't expose the treated area to the sun during the period of your treatment and for a few weeks thereafter. Use a sunblock of medium strength (7 to 8) on the treated area after this time.

A treated breast is usually somewhat firmer than normal. In most patients the breast remains the same size, but in some instances it may shrink or become larger. This is another reaction that varies from woman to woman.

Many women ask about the effect of radiation on their immune system. It has been found that immunological changes as a result of local radiation therapy have no bearing on the course of cancer, nor have we found changes in immunity to other diseases.

Does Radiation Exposure Ever Cause Cancer?

Under certain conditions there have been radiation-induced cancers, but these are not the result of radiation therapy for breast cancer. The connection seems to have to do with the radiation dose and the age of the person who is exposed. People nineteen and younger are at the highest risk for radiation-induced cancer. After thirty-five, the risk is negligible.

The incidence of radiation-induced malignancies increases with an increase in dose up to a range of three hundred to one thousand rads. Thereafter, the incidence decreases as the dose goes up.

At the lower doses, more normal cells are transformed into malignant cells. At the higher doses, cells that show malignant transformations are destroyed and the number of transformed cells actually goes down. In fact, when the radiation dose reaches therapeutic range—more than 4,500 rads—the risk is negligible.

Women at Hiroshima, particularly young women, who had been exposed to radiation from the atomic bomb had an increased incidence of breast cancer. The level of radiation they received was three to four hundred rads, and about sixty to seventy women per one hundred thousand developed breast cancer. In the un-irradiated population the rate was about twenty-five per one hundred thousand.

In the past, women who had many fluoroscopic examinations for tuberculosis had a higher incidence of breast cancer. Each examination delivered four to twenty rads and many women received more than one hundred fluoroscopies. Such women had an eighty percent higher incidence of breast cancer than the general population.

There is a similar situation among women who were treated for postpartum mastitis with radiation doses of one hundred to six hundred rads.

What is the connection between these statistics and the treatment of breast cancer? Radiation therapy after lumpectomy uses at least 4,500 rads. There has been no increased breast cancer observed either in the treated or in the opposite breasts of women who received this treatment. The incidence of new cancers in the opposite breast is the same for women who received radiotherapy as for those treated with mastectomy alone.

Radiation Therapy After Recurrence

Once we have treated a breast with radiation, we can seldom use this treatment again. If there is a local recurrence, further surgery and chemotherapy probably will be the treatments of choice.

Surgery and radiation therapy are the essential partners in breast conservation. The track record of this two-pronged attack on cancer is remarkably good.

9

PROGNOSIS

~❦~

Whether you had a lumpectomy followed by a course of radiation, or a mastectomy without radiation, you have now reached the point at which you and your doctors must plan the next strategy.

Cancer—an enemy if ever there was one—has been beaten back, but we want to make certain it stays that way. The first step to achieving that goal is to ask a simple question: Should we now use further therapy to prevent the recurrence or spread of the cancer?

For most physicians, the answer depends on the patient's prognosis, her prospect of recovery, and continued good health. Decisions about using chemotherapy and hormone therapy are often made on the basis of prognosis.

To use a military analogy, the more powerful the enemy, the

further our intelligence service tells us he has advanced against us, the more powerful must be the force we use against him. Moreover, since we are fighting in our own home territory, we have to eliminate him without destroying ourselves.

DETERMINING THE RISK OF RECURRENCE

How do we look into the future and arrive at a prognosis? On the basis of risk factors, individual criteria that we examine in each patient to determine what the likelihood is that she will remain disease-free. Each of these factors gives us some information about the future, and taken together, they can provide some guidance to the physician about what treatment is most apt to be helpful.

No one knows for sure the risk of recurrence of any particular cancer for any particular person. We only know statistically that given such and such circumstance, in a group of patients, such and such is likely to happen if the disease is untreated.

But even after the most exhaustive analysis of risk factors, scientists have had to concede that there are more individual questions than there are general conclusions. When we say, "Here is the prognosis for someone with three cancerous lymph nodes and a two-centimeter invasive breast tumor," we're really saying, "Here is the pattern of consequences that we've observed in a lot of people who were in that situation." We cannot say to any particular person, "This is what's going to happen to you."

Why then do we want to assess any one person's risk factors? Because many people believe that these may provide guidance as to the next treatment to use. But the fact is that even when we consider risk factors in the light of making treatment decisions, their impact is fairly limited. We've seen that surgery is the primary treatment for almost all breast cancer. We've seen that if the surgery choice is lumpectomy, the next treatment is radiation. When we get into the heart of the next chapter, on chemotherapy and hormone therapy, you will also see that there is fairly consistent agreement in most instances on what steps must be taken next.

Only a few gray areas remain, circumstances in which there are questions about whether or not to use chemotherapy and hormone therapy and what the specific regimens should be. It is in these situations that determining prognosis becomes especially important.

We evaluate prognosis primarily by the stage of the cancer (see Chapter Three), the combination of factors by which the extent of the illness is defined. Those primary factors are

- infiltration
- size of tumor
- lymph-node involvement

Let's now propose an unthinkable question: Suppose we did the surgery, and perhaps the radiation, but we chose to do no chemotherapy or hormone therapy, whatever the patient's condition might be? What would the recurrence and survival statistics be, given a particular tumor size, a particular degree of infiltration, a particular number of involved lymph nodes? What risk factors would point to a favorable or unfavorable outcome?

Infiltration

As we saw in Chapter Three, cancers can be *in situ*, that is, confined to their site of origin. When they have broken through the wall of the duct or lobule, they are said to have infiltrated— that is, they have spread to the local area or to a distant site in the body.

The risk of recurrence of an *in situ* cancer after mastectomy is almost zero. With infiltrating cancers, the size of the tumor is important, but risk is also related to the pattern of infiltration. For example, cancer in the lymphatics of the breast itself is not as significant as the involvement of the lymphatics of the skin or, as very rarely happens, involvement of the chest muscle. These latter cancers are more likely to spread to other parts of the body, no matter what the size of the primary tumor.

As we will see in the chapter on chemotherapy and hormone therapy, infiltration is often the risk factor that determines whether or not we will recommend further treatment.

Tumor Size

The larger the tumor, the higher the risk of recurrence of cancer, either within the breast, in the local area, or at a distant site. If there were no further treatment, and if the nodes were negative, here are the statistical chances—depending upon tumor size— that five years after diagnosis the patient would be cancer-free:

- Less than one centimeter (about three-eighths of an inch): more than ninety percent cancer-free.
- Up to two centimeters (about three-fourths of an inch): seventy-five percent cancer-free.
- Two to five centimeters (about three-fourths of an inch to about two inches): thirty to forty percent cancer-free.
- Five centimeters (about two inches) or larger: twenty-five percent cancer-free.

Lymph-Node Involvement

There is some correlation between tumor size and the likelihood of lymph-node involvement. In a group of patients with tumors smaller than one centimeter, a little over twenty percent had some cancerous lymph nodes. Among patients whose tumors were larger than five centimeters, sixty percent had lymph-node involvement.

We get our first decisive information about the lymph nodes in the armpit after breast surgery when, as we saw on pages 113–115, they are removed and examined. These nodes provide us with information vital to evaluating the disease.

As to the influence of node involvement on the recurrence of cancer, in general:

- The more nodes involved, the greater the risk, with the highest risk among patients who have ten or more cancerous nodes.
- The larger any tumor in the nodes, the greater the risk.
- If the tumor breaks through the capsule of the node and

154

spreads to surrounding tissue, the risk of recurrence increases.

As we have seen, the lymph nodes are grouped in three levels, from those that extend from the top of the breast to those high up in the armpit. Five-year survival, in one study (in which treatment was limited to surgery), was sixty-five percent when Level I nodes were involved, forty-five percent when Level II nodes were involved, and only twenty percent for women whose disease had spread high in the armpit to the Level III nodes.

OTHER RISK FACTORS

Hormone Receptor Levels

We discussed the question of whether tumors are hormone-receptor positive or negative on pages 86–87. These findings affect the prognosis.

Cells can be classified by whether they are mature (differentiated) or immature (undifferentiated). In general, mature cells are not very good at dividing and multiplying, but they do specialized work very efficiently, and they produce large numbers of estrogen and progesterone receptors.

The less mature a cell, the less likely it is to have hormone receptors on its surface and the greater its ability to divide and multiply. If immature cells are normal, they will develop into mature cells and take on their characteristics. But when cancer is present, it arrests these cells in the course of their maturation process, sometimes before they have developed the ability to produce hormone receptors.

There is a modest improvement in outlook if both estrogen and progesterone receptors can be detected in the tumor. Women with one or the other of the receptors have an intermediate advantage. Those with tumors that have no receptors are at a somewhat higher risk of recurrence. As an indicator of prognosis, the presence or absence of hormone receptors is much less significant than the size of the tumor or the number of nodes involved.

155

The Genetic Material of the Cells

Chapter Five, on pathology, described a test called flow cytometry, which is used to examine the DNA of the cells to determine whether there is a normal or abnormal number of chromosomes. We know that tumor cells have lost their ability to fully control chromosome duplication so that instead of the normal two copies of each chromosome (diploid), a cancerous cell may have fewer or more chromosome copies (aneuploid).

The most favorable outcome for breast cancer is usually when cell populations are diploid. When there are fewer or more chromosomes in a cell population, the risk of a recurrence of cancer increases two to three times.

The S phase is the period in which the cell is synthesizing DNA in preparation for dividing. Flow cytometry is one of the tests that can tell us how many cells in a given population are in the S phase at the time of the test. Many laboratories consider that if more than seven percent of cells are in this phase, this is an unfavorable risk factor. Patients with diploid tumors and a small number of S-phase cells have a ninety percent five-year survival rate.

Other tests measure actual cell proliferation. Though the terms and methods of measurement differ from test to test, in general, the fewer cells proliferating, the smaller the risk. In one test, when eighteen percent or more of the cell population is proliferating, that is considered high risk.

In the past few years we have learned that the presence and heightened activity of certain genes, called oncogenes, is associated with the capacity for more vigorous cell growth. The presence of one of these genes is now considered a risk factor for the recurrence of breast cancer. This gene goes by several names, which you may hear from any one of your team of doctors: HER-2/neu, erbB-2.

Whatever it is called, it has been discovered that an increased number of copies of this gene may be produced in breast cancer. The more copies, the more serious the prognosis.

Another gene that may limit growth in normal cells is the suppressor gene p53 (see page 259). Overproduction of abnormal, improperly functioning protein by this gene is associated with a less favorable prognosis. In normal breast cells, the production of an enzyme called cathepsin D is controlled by estrogen. Though this is a fairly new discovery that remains to be investigated further, we do know that in node-negative tumors—which normally indicate a good outlook—high levels of cathepsin D seem to be an indicator of a poor prognosis.

What can we make of all this arcane information? How can we use such data for any particular patient to decide whether the risk of a recurrence of cancer warrants the use of chemotherapy and hormone therapy?

Well, from my point of view, you can't hang your hat on any one of these factors. First of all, there are a lot of complexities. For example:

- Small tumors are better than large tumors, aren't they? Not if there's lymph-node involvement. That might indicate that even though the tumor is still small, it's vigorous enough to have already spread to the nodes.
- If the diploid situation is good, that means a good prognosis, doesn't it? Perhaps not, if the S phase is high. But, in another twist, if the lymph nodes are negative, the prognosis is quite favorable.

The fact is that most women who have had breast cancer now receive chemotherapy or hormone therapy. Almost the only exceptions are those who had very small, non-invasive cancers. The question of whether or not to give further treatment remains open only for women with the very smallest invasive tumors, negative axillary nodes, or an extremely slight amount of infiltration.

Many physicians depend on risk factors to make a decision in those cases, but it seems to me that at the moment, the ground is still too slippery to do so. Perhaps in a few years, after we've had a better chance to see how these factors prove themselves, we'll be able to use them as prognosticators. At the moment, it is still far from clear that they can be the basis on which to determine further treatment. Occasionally you may see laboratory reports referring to findings as "favorable" or "unfavorable." Given the uncertainty of how to sum up the significance of the lesser prognostic tests, whose results are often contradictory, such simplified interpretations are misleading. For instance, *in situ* cancers (see page 86), if tested, frequently are associated with poor risk factors, yet the cure rate for this form of breast cancer is close to 100 percent.

So, though we are getting a lot more sophisticated information now than we have ever had before, we do not yet have clear correlations. For that reason, it is my view that we should collect as much evidence as we can and do thorough research to measure the impact of what we are learning. But in the meantime, when there is any doubt about where the prognosis is pointing, we should use preventive therapy. As the next chapter indicates, it is far better to err on the side of safety than to regret later not having used all the weapons at our command.

10

PREVENTIVE HORMONE THERAPY AND CHEMOTHERAPY

❧

Y ou have come through breast surgery and perhaps a
course of radiation therapy, and now your surgeon may
be telling you that the next step to be considered is
chemotherapy or hormone therapy. No wonder many
women throw up their hands and say, "Enough! The cancer's
gone. I don't want any more treatment and I certainly don't want
anything done to me that's going to make my hair fall out."

This chapter will explain the lifesaving usefulness of chemotherapy and hormone therapy, the treatment processes, the details of the drug regimens that may be suggested for you, their
side effects and benefits, and how you evaluate whether these
therapies are right for you.

WHY CHEMOTHERAPY AND/OR HORMONE THERAPY?

Why should you even consider systemic treatment, treatment with drugs that circulate throughout your body? After all, your surgeon has probably assured you that he has removed all the cancer.

Chemotherapy and/or hormone therapy is being considered because there is a possibility that the cancer has traveled to other parts of the body, even though there may be no discernible evidence of this. Surgery has greatly reduced the risk that the cancer will spread, but some risk does remain, as we discussed in the previous chapter. Systemic therapy is used to bring us as close as we can now get to eliminating that risk.

Removing the breast, as we have seen, cures *in situ* cancer. In the case of infiltrating cancer—breast cancer that has moved outside the duct or lobule in which it originated—even though it may still appear to be confined to the breast, we cannot be certain that it has not spread to other parts of the body.

Systemic therapy interferes with the growth and spread of cancer. It is often referred to as adjuvant therapy, because it is used to supplement the effectiveness of surgery. Unlike surgery or radiation, systemic treatment, because it travels through the bloodstream, acts against cancer in distant sites and significantly reduces the risk of recurrence. In fact, it can reduce that risk by up to one-third and it can markedly affect the life span of women who have had breast cancer.

But, to get that result, treatment must begin fairly soon, with what I describe to my patients as "due, deliberate speed." Despite the natural reluctance of most people to undertake still another course of therapy after surgery and possibly radiation, adjuvant therapy isn't something you can postpone. You can't say, "Okay. You've convinced me. The next time I get sick I'll do it."

To put it plainly, waiting until there is a problem reduces the effectiveness of systemic treatment; it is much more powerful an adversary against cancer when it is brought to bear against what is called subclinical disease, disease that is so limited that we cannot find it through the usual tests available to us.

This may sound like medical voodoo and it is logical to ask, "If you can't find it, how do you know you've cured it? Maybe it wasn't there in the first place."

We know it was there from statistical evidence that has accumulated since 1975 in studies of large numbers of women in various regions of the United States as well as abroad. These data show that the recurrence of cancer for patients at relatively high risk, as well as for those whose risk is much lower, can be significantly reduced by early intervention with hormone therapy or chemotherapy.

WHO SHOULD GET CHEMOTHERAPY AND/OR HORMONE THERAPY?

For women with breast cancer, it is in the use of chemotherapy that most of the complex questions and choices among options arise. There is considerable controversy about which patients should receive chemotherapy and what mix of drugs should be used; if hormones should be administered; and whether such treatment should be routine for all women who have had breast cancer. Much of this difference of opinion has to do with:

- the size of the tumor
- whether the disease has spread to the lymph nodes
- whether you were pre- or postmenopausal at the time the tumor appeared

In general:

- Chemotherapy works best in premenopausal women.
- Hormone therapy works best for postmenopausal women, particularly those whose tumors were estrogen- or progesterone-receptor positive. (See pages 86–87.)

BUT

- We are learning that, combined with hormone therapy, chemotherapy may have a place in the treatment of postmenopausal women, though its precise role is still under study.

161

- Similarly, there seem to be circumstances where the use of hormone therapy combined with chemotherapy in premenopausal women may be appropriate. More work remains to be done to clarify its use.

Though we will come back to these questions at the end of this chapter, it may be simpler to begin by looking at the question this way: If you had an infiltrating cancer, most physicians at this time will recommend preventive chemotherapy and/or hormone therapy, unless the tumor was very small. (Some of us believe that *any* infiltrating cancer, whatever the size of the tumor, should be treated with preventive systemic therapy.)

You should follow that recommendation for the following reasons:

- No one dies of cancer in the breast, only of cancer that has spread outside the breast.
- Systemic chemotherapy and hormone therapy can prevent the spread of cancer.
- Chemotherapy and hormone therapy are saving tens of thousands of lives, particularly of women with an average risk of recurrence.
- Women who in the past had no chance even to survive, now have the possibility of cure.

Why, if those things are true, aren't women rushing enthusiastically to systemic therapy? We all know the answer. People are terrified of the side effects. They do not want to be nauseated, or lose their hair, or gain weight. For women who have just had breast surgery, the threat of further cosmetic assault and physical discomfort is almost unbearable. Many women are as terrified of chemotherapy as they are of the consequences of not taking the treatment.

We will discuss side effects in greater detail as this chapter proceeds, but there are a few reassuring amulets you can carry with you through these pages:

- The drugs used in systemic therapy are not poison. In general, used prudently, they destroy bad cells, spare good cells.

- Most side effects will pass relatively quickly. They are not permanent.
- A good physician can ameliorate the most feared side effects.

WHO IS THE RIGHT PHYSICIAN?

The first task, as in every phase of illness, is to find a good physician to administer chemotherapy or hormone therapy. Luckily, you are not starting from scratch. In most instances, your surgeon regularly refers patients to one or two physicians whom he has worked with and whom he trusts.

Even so, cautions are necessary. Here are the qualifications you should look for:

- The chemotherapist should be board-certified or board-eligible in medical oncology, the medical treatment of tumors, particularly malignant tumors. That is, she should have completed a fellowship in this specialty and then passed an exhaustive examination. (Board-eligible or, as it is sometimes called, board-qualified, specialists have taken their training but not the examinations.)
- Alternatively, the chemotherapist may be a hematologist. She should be board-certified or board-qualified in hematology, the study of the blood and its disorders.
- She should have extensive experience and skill in the treatment of breast cancer.
- She should be someone you can comfortably relate to.

> *Chemotherapy can be dangerous. Do not accept treatment from a surgeon or local physician just because he says he can do it. Expertise in the use of these techniques is essential.*

A COMPANION

You will find it especially helpful to have with you during at least your first visits to the chemotherapist someone who knows you well and with whom you feel comfortable. Though you will probably find that the treatment is less traumatic than what you may have been dreading, for the first few times take your personal advocate, a friend, or a family member with you to help you raise questions with the doctor, to remember what he said, or simply to provide a supportive presence.

THE PHYSICIAN'S OFFICE

Though this is not something that came up in our discussions of the qualifications of other doctors, the physical arrangement of the oncologist's office is particularly important. This is not a matter of interior design; it is the reality that it is hard to treat patients with dignity unless there is room to treat them separately.

You should be given some privacy during your chemotherapy, and this is not really possible in a room where several people are receiving treatment at the same time.

THE PRETREATMENT EXAMINATION

During the initial visit, the physician will take a complete medical history and do a thorough physical examination. Make sure to take with you to that first appointment a list of the details of your medical history, as well as a list of *all* medications you are now taking, including vitamins. Make sure to note the dosages. You will also need the operative report, the pathology report, and the pathology slides. (See pages 224–225 for information on how to get these.) Before the visit, write down any questions you may have about why chemotherapy or hormone therapy is being recommended, and during the visit, raise any concerns you have about the effectiveness and side effects of the particular plan the doctor is proposing. You and she should discuss these matters thoroughly.

Optimally, you should be seen by the physician every time you go for a treatment. Her first questions will give her an overview of your general condition: How have you been feeling? What is your general condition like?

After that broad view, the doctor will explore with you the subtleties of your condition since your previous treatment:

- Appetite—Are you eating normally? Are there any foods you especially like or dislike?
- Energy level—Are you living your normal life? Do you go out? Go shopping? Go to work?
- Sleep—Are there changes in your normal sleep pattern? Do you fall asleep easily? Wake up at your normal time?
- Pain—Do you have any pain? Where exactly is it? How severe? Do you take any medication for it?
- The body systems are reviewed, including a discussion of symptoms such as headaches, sore throat, runny nose, earache, cough, sputum production, nausea, vomiting, diarrhea, constipation, or a burning sensation when you urinate.

By no means will you have all—or any—of these symptoms, nor will everything you may feel be a result of your treatment, but this is a time when you and the doctor want to know as precisely as possible what is going on in your body.

Each time you arrive for a treatment at the oncologist's office, a nurse or technician will prick your finger in order to take a blood count.

A brief physical examination is often done at every visit. It includes

- A breast examination for any gross changes
- A general examination that concentrates on nearby lymph nodes and the chest

At intervals, the doctor may order scans of your body, X rays, or other tests to monitor your condition, including any effects of the therapy. A more thorough general physical examination will also be conducted from time to time, as well as a very thorough palpation of the breasts.

At each visit you should review with the doctor any questions you may have; as always, write these down beforehand so that you don't forget to ask them. This question period helps crystallize information about your general condition; it can also be a chance for you and the doctor to pick up on anything that may have been missed during the last visit.

As in the description of other procedures, all this may sound formidable. The truth is, it takes almost as long to describe as to do. In fact, the entire examination and discussions during your treatment visits should take only fifteen to twenty minutes. They are, however, a vital aspect of the treatment itself and an important reassurance to you that you are getting careful and concerned attention.

THE TREATMENT

We will begin this section with certain general information on the use of adjuvant chemotherapy for patients who have had breast cancer. The mechanics of treatment may differ from doctor to doctor. As noted above, make sure you discuss the treatment your oncologist plans for you in detail, and that you understand and feel comfortable with it. Raise any questions you now have and continue to do this if other concerns arise later.

How Are the Drugs Administered?

While some chemotherapy drugs are taken by mouth, most are given intravenously, that is, directly into a vein. This can be done by starting an intravenous infusion (IV) of dextrose and water and then administering the drug by adding it to the IV.

It can also be done by an injection of the undiluted medication directly into a vein—usually at the top of the hand. This is called a direct push, and it is a very simple way to administer the drugs. It spares the patient from waiting the thirty minutes or so that it takes for an infusion to be completed.

Who Administers the Drugs?

It takes a very skilled, experienced person to administer either an infusion or a direct-push injection. Women often worry about whether chemotherapy causes a "breakdown" of the veins. That is not a common occurrence if those administering the drugs are good at what they do. The proper needle must be used and the patient should press on the spot where the needle was placed for five minutes after the treatment is completed.

Usually the person who gives the treatment is a specially trained and sometimes certified oncology nurse. She knows how to insert the needle in the vein without damaging it. She also knows how to test that it is actually in the vein before administering the injection itself. This is important if we are to prevent leakage under the skin, which can cause problems with certain cytotoxic drugs.

Will They Have to Poke Around to Find a Vein?

In most cases, there is no problem in locating a good site for the injection. In instances when women have more body fat or very tiny veins, however, it can be more difficult to "find" the vein. In such cases, it may be necessary to tap the skin to bring the vein up toward the surface. If you think you require special attention and that the person who is treating you does not have that level of expertise, speak up. The physician has probably done many thousands of such injections over the years, and, when it is necessary, you should have the most experienced hands available to you. It is reassuring to know, however, that in some patients who have required long-term therapy, drugs have been administered for years without discomfort.

Are There Other Ways to Administer Chemotherapy?

In some situations, plastic tubing is inserted under the skin and connected to one of the larger veins leading to the heart. This is a surgical procedure that is performed in the hospital, and the device remains in place after it has been inserted.

In the Hickman or the Broviac device of this type, the tubing comes out through the skin and ends in a cylinder with a rubber diaphragm, into which medication can be directly injected.

In the Infus-a-Port and other similar devices, the entry to the tubing is via a flat, buttonlike port, about the size of a nickel, under the skin. The needle must go through the skin into this port each time an injection is given.

Generally speaking, such apparatus is not necessary in order to avoid vein "breakdown." Ordinarily, with care, the vein will not be damaged. And though they may seem a convenient way to administer intravenous medication, these devices can cause problems:

- They have to be surgically implanted.
- They can be a source of infection.
- They must be flushed regularly with an anticoagulant to prevent them from becoming clogged.

Very occasionally, there are compelling reasons for the use of these tubing devices. A woman may not tolerate repeated injections into a small vein. Sometimes there may be swelling in the arm that makes access to the vein difficult. And some people prefer the ready access to their veins that such devices provide.

On balance, of course, this choice is an individual matter, but something else needs to be considered: the patient should feel that when she leaves the office, she is fine. In the office, she is, unavoidably, a patient. When she leaves, she is a normal person who can go about her business normally. It is hard for many people to see themselves in this way with plastic tubing embedded in their chests.

THE DRUGS

The hormones used in hormone therapy for breast cancer normally play a role in regulating breast cell growth and survival. When they are given therapeutically, they cause dramatic shrinking of breast tumors, without damaging cells in the rest of the body.

Drugs used for chemotherapy are called cytotoxic, meaning that they act largely by destroying cells. The question that inevitably comes up now is this: Won't cytotoxic drugs destroy normal cells, too?

When properly administered, cytotoxic drugs will kill some normal cells, but not many. The drugs used in chemotherapy are useful because cancer cells are much more sensitive to their effects than are normal cells. It is this difference in sensitivity that is the edge we utilize to treat the cancer without injuring the patient.

Dosage

In the preventive treatment of breast cancer, most women are given more or less the same dose of hormones by mouth, twice a day. Tamoxifen (Nolvadex), the hormone most commonly used, is given in a daily dose of twenty mgs.

In chemotherapy, on the other hand, dosage is individually tailored to each patient, in order to give the highest dose possible that will kill the cancer cells and not harm her. If the dose is too low, the cancer cells will not be destroyed. If the dose is too high, the side effects will not be acceptable.

Though there may seem to be high-dose and low-dose advocates among oncologists, in fact, the dosage range that is effective as well as tolerated is fairly narrow. However, the schedule as well as the dosage is important in administering these drugs. Cancer cells can be sensitive to chemotherapy in some stages of their growth and resistant to it in others. What is *not* possible is to give a single dose so high that it kills all cancer cells at one time. That level of dosage cannot be tolerated. The higher the dose, the less frequently it can be given; the lower the dose, the more frequently.

There are various programs of chemotherapy: weekly, bi-weekly, every three weeks, and others. The frequency will vary with the program, with the drugs used, and with the doses. Despite these variations, there is one very important strategy in using chemotherapy to fight cancer: *hit hard as early in the course of the disease as possible*.

That doesn't mean we should load the patient up with a megadose of the most aggressive drugs available. But neither does it make sense to "lead up to" the program that will eventually be used. The physician should make careful plans about the drugs that will be used, how they will be combined, their dosages, and the schedule—and then go to it.

This approach works best because there is reason to believe that not only does the number of tumor cells increase as the disease progresses, but so does the possibility that cells will develop that will be resistant to chemotherapy. For that reason, we should act vigorously from the start.

Timing

Preventive hormone therapy should begin within four weeks of surgery. Studies in patients whose tumor was confined to the breast at the time of surgery (Stage I, see page 41) indicate that tamoxifen should be given for a period of five years. Taking tamoxifen beyond five years provides no additional benefit. However, until the results of ongoing studies are available for those at higher risk because of extension of the tumor to nearby lymph nodes, it seems prudent to continue this therapy for a longer period of time.

Adjuvant chemotherapy should also begin about four weeks following surgery. If you need both radiation (see Chapter Eight) and chemotherapy, the sequence of the treatments will vary depending on the individual situation. Radiation can be given before, during, or after chemotherapy. The optimal timing is now under study.

As to duration of chemotherapy, we know that a single treatment does not destroy every cancer cell. Our goal is to get rid of all cancer cells because even if 99.9 percent of the billions of cancer cells that were present were to be destroyed, the remaining .1 percent still would leave a significant number capable of multiplying and causing grave harm. We also know that because the drugs attack the DNA of multiplying cells, any one treatment may "miss" those cells that are not actively preparing to divide at that time. Like hibernating bears, these noncycling cells may awake later and become active.

For these and other reasons, repeated treatments of chemotherapy are used over a period of time that may vary from several months to half a year, or to one, two, or three years. The stage of the disease, the particular drugs that are used, and the risks are all taken into account in determining the duration of treatment.

Some oncologists believe that no program of preventive chemotherapy should extend for more than six months; but there is an interesting line of reasoning that may help in deciding how long chemotherapy should continue in some cases. We saw, a few paragraphs back, that when tamoxifen is used, an extended period of treatment is necessary and more than five years may be better for those at higher risk. The lesson to be learned from that pattern may be that for some patients, especially those who have more advanced disease when they come to us, adjuvant therapy may be effective in longer programs that employ innovative plans of drug intensity, intermittent administration, drug cycling, and other techniques discussed in the course of this chapter.

Combining Drugs

At the present time, using only one single drug against cancer simply isn't effective. Most modern chemotherapy programs for breast cancer combine at least three drugs and as many as six. We're not sure why this strategy works, but perhaps it is because cells that respond to one drug don't respond to another. By using several substances we get an overlapping effectiveness.

The Types of Drugs

There are four types of drugs currently in use for preventive treatment of breast cancer:

171

- **Alkylating agents,** the first group, damage the programs that control growth in the chromosomes of the tumor cells.
- **Antimetabolites,** the second group, interfere with the manufacture of nucleotides, the simple substances that make up DNA.
- **Natural products,** the third group, interfere with cell structure and cell division.
- **Hormones,** the fourth group, affect the growth of breast cancer cells.

ALKYLATING AGENTS

The most widely used alkylating agent is Cytoxan (cyclophosphamide). It can be given by mouth or intravenously, and it is not activated until it is processed in the liver.

Similar to Cytoxan is Thiotepa, a drug that requires very careful monitoring because it is highly toxic to bone marrow. It is given in very small doses intravenously.

A related but not typical alkylating product is Adriamycin (doxorubicin). This drug must be given intravenously, and it must be carefully administered since it can be extremely damaging to the skin if it leaks out of the vein.

ANTIMETABOLITES

Methotrexate and 5-fluorouracil are the two antimetabolites widely used for the treatment of breast cancer. In adjuvant treatment they are usually given intravenously.

Leucovorin, a vitamin derivative of folic acid, is sometimes used in combination with these drugs to modulate their activity. It may be given by mouth or intravenously.

NATURAL PRODUCTS

Vincristine (Oncovin) and vinblastine (Velban) are derived from the periwinkle plant. A chemically altered product of the same plant, vinorelbine (Navelbine), is also available. These work in tiny concentrations. Recent additions to this drug group are paclitaxel (Taxol) and docetaxal (Taxotere), whose original sources were respectively the barks of the Pacific and European yew trees. Taxol is now also produced synthetically. Given intravenously, all these drugs can cause damage if they accidentally leak into the skin.

HORMONE-RELATED SUBSTANCES

Prednisone, a drug related to cortisone, probably works in adjuvant therapy because, as a hormone, it enhances the effects of the other cytotoxic drugs. It may also have other antitumor properties.

Tamoxifen (Nolvadex), as noted, is the most widely used hormone-related drug. It is an antiestrogen or hormone antagonist because, though it is itself a weak estrogen, it interferes with the action of estrogen on cancer cells and inhibits tumor growth. It is given by mouth.

Halotestin (fluoxymesterone) is a male hormone preparation that is sometimes used in hormone-receptive patients to inhibit tumor growth.

How Are These Drugs Combined?

The following section is a brief survey of the way these drugs are combined in systemic therapy. You may want to read the material now or you may want to wait and use it as a reference when you and your physician discuss your planned treatment.

TAMOXIFEN

We begin with this hormone-related substance because it is so frequently used, often alone, sometimes in combination with other drugs. Several years ago there were some reports that seemed to indicate that tamoxifen interfered with the action of chemotherapy, and for that reason, the treatments were not used together. However, in 1984, a study was initiated of 1,200 women, age fifty or over, all of whom had lymph-node involvement and were also hormone-receptor positive (see pages 86–87). Reported on in 1990, this study revealed that there was significant benefit to women who received both tamoxifen and chemotherapy, compared with those who received tamoxifen alone. There was no evidence at all of an unfavorable reaction between the two treatments. They may, in fact, even augment each other.

CMF

CMF—Cytoxan, methotrexate, and 5-fluorouracil—is the proto-type chemotherapy combination because of its documented record of improving survival rates in several groups of women.

This is the most commonly used schedule for administering this combination of drugs:

- Cytoxan is taken daily, by mouth, for the first fourteen days of every four-week month (that is, every twenty-eight days, rather than the thirty or thirty-one days of a calendar month).
- The other two drugs, methotrexate and 5-fluorouracil, are given intravenously on the first and eighth days of the four-week month.

In a variant of this schedule, all three drugs are administered intravenously once every three weeks.

CMF is usually administered for six months. Studies of continuing this treatment program for up to two years have shown no additional benefits.

CAF

This program combines Cytoxan, Adriamycin, and 5-fluorouracil. It is administered on the first and eighth days of the four-week month, with no medication during the remaining two weeks of the month. Treatment usually continues for four to six months.

FAC

Similar to CAF, and using the same drugs, this program emphasizes somewhat higher doses of Adriamycin, generally on the first day of a twenty-eight-day cycle. Another program treats with all three drugs one day every three weeks.

Adria/CMF

A three-month program of high-dose Adriamycin is followed by six months of CMF. An alternative regimen consists of six months of CMFVP followed by three months of high-dose Adriamycin. This is used for patients with four or more positive nodes.

CMFVP

In this plan, vincristine and prednisone (or prednisolone, a similar drug) are added to CMF. This combination of drugs is used in my own practice once every week for six or twelve months, depending on the stage of the tumor at the time of surgery. The program is administered by some physicians for six to eight weeks on a weekly basis, and then for two out of four weeks. The duration of the treatment is usually from nine months to a year. There is evidence, though it is by no means conclusive, that CMFVP is more effective than CMF.

MF

This program combines methotrexate and 5-fluorouracil with the folic acid derivative leucovorin, and thus avoids the use of Cytoxan, which, as we will see, may have troublesome side effects. It has been effective in treating women with no lymph-node involvement.

Sequential High-Dose Therapy

High doses of single drugs such as Cytoxan, Adriamycin, and Taxol are given in close sequence. Since only one drug is used at a time, higher doses can be employed than if the same agents are used in combination.

Very-High-Dose Chemotherapy in Conjunction with Bone-Marrow and/or Stem-Cell Transplant

Though not yet established as a treatment for patients with advanced-stage breast cancer, people who have blood-related cancers like leukemia and lymphoma have been treated in recent years with doses of chemotherapy so large that they destroy not only cancer cells but normal bone-marrow cells as well. After this treatment, patients have no residual bone marrow to produce the white blood cells that protect against infection or the platelets that prevent bleeding.

In order to counteract this effect, before such chemotherapy the patient's own bone marrow is removed from the body and stored. In addition, drugs are used to stimulate the patient's marrow to produce large numbers of immature white blood cells that are released into the circulating bloodstream. These "stem cells" are also removed and stored. After very-high-dose chemotherapy is completed, the bone marrow and/or stem cells are given back to the patient.

Such programs, administered in combination with high-dose alkylating agents, have recently become available for breast cancer patients. Autologous (meaning from the patient's own body) transplants are now being increasingly used as adjuvant treatment for patients at highest risk for recurrence. While this treatment remains in the experimental stage, the promising results seen to date have made such therapy a widely used alternative for those with ten or more involved lymph nodes. Studies in progress will establish whether the long-term benefits of such treatments warrant their greater toxicity.

These procedures now cost about one hundred thousand dollars, and insurance companies are often resistant to paying for what they consider experimental treatments, regardless of the illness. The recent introduction of drugs such as colony-stimulating factors is helping to hasten recovery from bone-marrow and stem-cell transplantation and thereby cut costs by about one-third; but only if and when the procedure becomes an approved form of therapy for breast cancer is the insurance situation likely to change.

General Side Effects

Hormone therapy does not have especially troublesome side effects. Such side effects are the aspect of chemotherapy treatment that concerns patients most. The concern is valid, but

- Chemotherapy does have side effects, but they are usually transitory.

176

- Several side effects cause particular difficulty right after treatment, but they soon fade.
- There is no way to avoid side effects completely, but an experienced and careful physician can alleviate many of the adverse symptoms.

PAIN?

There is usually no pain associated with the administration of chemotherapy. Very occasionally, the drug may feel cold as it goes into the vein, but that feeling rarely lasts for more than a few seconds.

NAUSEA

Nausea is, for most of us, one of the most unpleasant of physical sensations. For that reason, apprehensiveness about nausea is sometimes worse than the actuality.

Most drugs do not cause immediate nausea unless a particularly large dose is being used and it is being pushed into the vein very fast. If you feel queasy during the treatment, mention it at once, and ask that the procedure be done more slowly.

Though this is not always the case, as we will see below, nausea is often a result of excessive acid secretion in the stomach caused by certain of the drugs. This nausea can be controlled with the use of preparations like Maalox, Tagamet, or Zantac. Eating a bowl of oatmeal can also be a help in settling your stomach.

Especially with the use of higher doses of chemotherapy, nausea may be severe enough to make it necessary for the doctor to prescribe a medication to reduce this symptom before beginning treatment. Until recently, the drugs available for this purpose, such as Compazine and Reglan, provided only modest relief and were associated with significant side effects of their own. While these medications are still useful for milder forms of nausea, a new category of drugs has recently been introduced, represented by Zofran and Kytril. These are available in both intravenous and oral preparations and have almost eliminated the immediate nausea associated with many forms of chemotherapy. When nausea persists for a day or two after treatment, it

177

can be treated at home with Compazine, Zofran, or Kytril taken by mouth. The last two drugs are very expensive, which has limited their use.

HAIR LOSS

This is the side effect that causes women the greatest sadness. At a time when they are extremely vulnerable, their appearance may be radically changed, and their illness given a visible and very upsetting public manifestation.

True. But . . . *every strand of hair will grow back.*

With that fact in mind, let's examine the question of hair loss.

With very high doses of Adriamycin, temporary hair loss cannot be prevented as of this writing. You should therefore arrange to buy an attractive hairpiece at the start of your treatment so that it will be on hand for the temporary period when you have lost your hair. Try to get one that is close, not only to your own color, but also to your own hair style, so that you will not have to cope with a new image of yourself when you look in the mirror.

With vincristine or lower doses of Adriamycin, we can prevent hair loss in women under sixty—and prevent or reduce it in women over sixty—by the use of a kind of tourniquet around the head during treatment. A narrow blood-pressure cuff, this band is set to an individualized pressure. The headband does not keep all of the drug from the scalp, but it does prevent the highest levels of the drug from reaching it. This precaution preserves the hair, and there has been no indication that it reduces the benefits of adjuvant therapy.

With vincristine and lower doses of Adriamycin, hair loss may also be ameliorated by using an ice pack on the head for fifteen minutes before and fifteen to thirty minutes after treatment.

FATIGUE

High doses of chemotherapy can cause a great deal of fatigue, especially on the first day after treatment. You should, however, feel little fatigue after a couple of days, though occasionally you may feel tired late in the day. If you do continue to feel exhausted, or if you have days when you are what some patients call "zonked out," tell the oncologist. If you are disabled or unable to function at a reasonable level, your drug dose is probably too high.

If you are extremely tired the first day or two after treatment, you should rest, but as soon as possible try to resume your normal level of activity. Many women find they can continue to work, though they may need some flexibility in their hours and schedules.

OTHER SIDE EFFECTS

Although relatively infrequent now, infection can be a problem with chemotherapy because most anticancer drugs affect bone marrow and, therefore, the production of the white blood cells the body uses to fight infection. This is one of the reasons you have a blood count taken every time you go for treatment. If there is a problem with your white-blood-cell count, your therapy will be adjusted. A colony-stimulating factor (a hormone that stimulates white-blood-cell growth) such as Neupogen may be prescribed to help restore white-blood-cell levels to normal more quickly. If you develop a fever, report it to your doctor.

The platelets are the cellular component of the blood that prevents bleeding. Since chemotherapy can affect the number of platelets, we must stop or postpone chemotherapy when these regular blood counts show the platelets to be at levels well above those associated with bleeding. You should also avoid taking aspirin, because it interferes with platelet function. The natural growth factor (thrombopoietin) for cells that are the source of platelets has been purified, and is now being used in clinical studies. First results are very promising, and this new drug should be available soon.

The term *phlebitis*, as we saw, describes an inflammation of the vein as well as the formation of a blood clot. It occurs infrequently in the legs as a side effect of chemotherapy, but it must be promptly treated.

Weight gain is a common and often unavoidable side effect of several of the drug programs. Ironically, many women about to undergo a course of chemotherapy are afraid that they are going to grow thin and gaunt; instead, they find that the opposite has happened.

The discomfort of the excess acid in the stomach that some

179

drugs cause can be mistaken for hunger. Sometimes, also, women eat because they are nauseated; still others seem to gain weight whether they eat more or not. Try to follow a sensible and weight-controlling diet, but don't chastise yourself for putting on a few pounds and don't go on a radical diet while you are on chemotherapy. If needed, your physician may prescribe drugs that reduce acid production. Eat nutritious and attractive food and remember that "this too shall pass." Most women go back to their normal weight six months to one year after chemotherapy.

Some people develop arthritis when chemotherapy is discontinued. It is a condition that will gradually disappear, usually within a year after its onset.

Sweating and "hot flashes" similar to those some women experience during menopause are among the general side effects of chemotherapy or hormone therapy. This symptom can be partially relieved by the use of a drug called Bellergal-S.

You may stop menstruating during systemic therapy, though you should not rely on this occurrence for contraception. Whether your period resumes depends on your age. Younger women are more likely to return to a normal menstrual cycle. Women in their forties and those closer to menopause are less likely to begin menstruating again.

Fertility, of course, is closely related to this. When your period returns, the likelihood is that you will again be able to conceive. And though couples quite naturally worry about this, there is no evidence that chemotherapy or hormone therapy causes either mutation to the eggs or birth defects.

Specific Drug-Related Side Effects

In addition to the general symptoms we've been reviewing, the following side effects, specific to particular drugs, can occur.

Remember: you may experience only a few—or even none—of these symptoms during the course of your treatment. Side effects can often be controlled by well-regulated dosages and schedules.

PREDNISONE

Like other cortisone products, this drug can cause emotional ups and downs, weight gain, insomnia, ulcers, and an elevation of blood-sugar levels. If given daily, the drug is most commonly used for a course of treatment lasting no more than eight weeks. For longer therapy, it is much better tolerated if it is taken every other day rather than daily. Prednisolone, a closely related preparation, has similar side effects.

TAMOXIFEN

Tamoxifen has relatively few significant side effects in most patients. An occasional person will have mild nausea or weight gain, and younger women may have annoying menopausal symptoms while they are taking the drug. Very rarely, a woman may notice some light facial hair growth as a result of using tamoxifen. Because it is itself a weak estrogen, the drug does not cause the loss of bone calcium associated with low estrogen levels. In fact, there is reason to believe tamoxifen helps prevent osteoporosis and heart disease caused by aging, and lowers blood cholesterol levels.

As to gynecological symptoms, a slight vaginal discharge is common. Tamoxifen, like estrogens used for hormone replacement therapy after menopause, modestly increases the risk of developing endometrial cancer. You should therefore see a gynecologist regularly.

HALOTESTIN

Facial hair growth, menstrual irregularities, deepening of the voice, and other masculinization may be associated with the use of this drug, though these changes are often mild and are reversible when the drug is stopped.

ADRIAMYCIN

Because this potent drug has so many side effects, it is not a front-line medication for low-risk breast cancer patients. If it is given in high doses at three- or four-week intervals, as it may be in CAF and FAC, Adriamycin can have a toxic effect on the heart, causing potentially significant heart muscle damage. When the total dose exceeds 750 to 1,000 mgs, depending on the patient's size, the heart muscle must be carefully monitored. For that reason, optimal programs are designed to keep Adriamycin below that threshold. However, in special circumstances where the continued use of Adriamycin is advisable, a second drug, Zinecard, can also be given to reduce Adriamycin's effects on the heart and permit larger doses. With relatively low doses and weekly treatment, there is less chance of a heart muscle problem.

The urine may be slightly red immediately after an Adriamycin injection. This is no cause for concern. Hair loss, nausea, vomiting, and inflammation of the mouth lining are also associated with the use of this drug. There can be marked skin damage if the drug infiltrates during injection.

CYTOXAN

The end products of Cytoxan, after it has been "used" by the body, can irritate the bladder and cause serious damage to the bladder wall. It is very important to increase your normal intake of water while you are using this drug; each doctor will have his own recommendations about how to accomplish this. For instance, you may be told to drink three glasses of water in addition to your normal intake within three hours of receiving Cytoxan. Ample water intake is especially important in hot weather. In certain individuals, Cytoxan can cause leukemia, but, after fifteen years of use, no increased incidence of leukemia has been seen in breast cancer patients on preventive chemotherapy.

CMFVP

Patients receiving this drug combination may develop persistent elevated temperature and a mild cough that may indicate a serious infection. Report any fever to your chemotherapist as soon as possible so that he can prescribe specific antibiotics.

5-FLUOROURACIL

This drug can cause irritation of the lining of the mouth and of the intestinal tract.

If mouth irritation occurs, avoid using commercial mouthwashes that may contain alcohol or other irritants. Rinse your mouth twice a day with one-eighth of a teaspoon of baking soda dissolved in a glass of lukewarm water. Brush your teeth gently and use a soft brush. This irritation is rarely severe, but numbing agents are available if they are necessary.

If severe diarrhea becomes a problem, the treatment must be stopped, though this usually occurs only at high doses, or in the case of somewhat lower doses of 5-fluorouracil when given in combination with leucovorin.

There may be a mild, reversible darkening of the skin after prolonged use of 5-fluorouracil.

METHOTREXATE

This drug may cause soreness of the mouth and diarrhea. In addition, nausea and vomiting may occur and methotrexate may cause fat accumulation in the liver, but such changes are usually reversible once the drug is stopped.

VINCRISTINE

In large doses, this drug is only given for a short time, six to eight weeks. That is because it can cause nerve damage that is sometimes permanent and that may result in constipation, numbness and tingling in the hands, feet, and fingers, and a loss of reflexes in the legs. These symptoms are not common when, instead of high doses, low doses of vincristine are used over a longer period of time.

IS SYSTEMIC THERAPY THE RIGHT STEP?

Let's begin with some general statements:

The purpose of chemotherapy or hormone therapy is to prevent the recurrence of cancer. That no one would choose to go through the experience of breast cancer more than once goes without saying. But there is another reality to be faced: it is extremely difficult to cure a recurrence. For that reason, the current consensus is that most patients with breast cancer should receive adjuvant therapy to prevent recurrence.

This point of view is particularly compelling because the side effects of adjuvant therapy are not life-threatening to the vast majority of patients. The most dangerous effects—heart muscle damage and the risk of infection—may occur in programs using Adriamycin, but only a very small percentage of women will be affected. Most side effects of adjuvant therapy are temporary and can be ameliorated by a carefully modulated program.

It is these considerations that have led me to the belief that adjuvant therapy should be used wherever there is an invasive cancer and therefore a risk of the disease's recurring. I think this is the most prudent policy. Moreover, it appears to be prudent even in circumstances where the risk is fairly small, as, for example, in the case of an invasive ductal cancer of less than one centimeter. I do not use chemotherapy or hormone therapy with intraductal or *in situ* lobular cancers where there is no lymph-node involvement and where the cancer has not spread outside the duct. I use adjuvant chemotherapy and/or hormone therapy for all other patients.

WHAT ADJUVANT THERAPY WILL I RECEIVE?

You will get different answers to that question from different on-cologists. That is because, as we have been learning in this chap-ter, there are many options to be considered as well as many risks.

When the oncologist proposes a program for you, she has to take into account what might be called the risk/benefit formula. If the disease has progressed far enough to put you at consider-able risk, the oncologist will be more likely to recommend "ag-gressive" treatment, despite the possible toxicity, if she thinks it will lead to long-lasting benefits. In such cases, the risk the cancer poses to survival needs to be weighed against the side effects of the treatment, though successful "aggressive" treat-ment does not necessarily have to be hard on the patient.

Tailoring Adjuvant Therapy to Risk

How do we tailor the treatment to the specific patient? First we determine her risk. Next we consider whether she is pre- or postmenopausal. Then we figure out from statistical evidence and from experience what has worked best for other women in this category.

When we are trying to decide what therapy is appropriate for a particular patient, we consider the following factors most important:

- invasion
- size of tumor
- lymph-node involvement

To review the general guidelines:

- Non-invasive *in situ* cancers have such a low risk of metastasizing that no chemotherapy is used. The role of hormone therapy is under investigation.

- If the tumor was primarily restricted to the inside of ducts or lobules (*in situ* cancer), but shows microscopic evidence of invasion, there is debate about whether chemotherapy or hormone therapy should be used.

- If the tumor is more invasive but is restricted to the breast and less than one centimeter in size, many oncologists give adjuvant therapy. Others feel that the risk for these women is too small to warrant using preventive therapy.

- If the tumor was invasive and one centimeter or more (about three-eighths of an inch) in diameter, preventive hormone therapy or chemotherapy is generally useful, whether or not the lymph nodes are involved.

- If the lymph nodes are involved, chemotherapy or hormone therapy should always be used, even if the tumor was less than one centimeter. There are differences of opinion only about how vigorous the treatment should be in correlation with the number of nodes involved.

THE RANGE OF TREATMENT

It would be wonderful if we had a simple, logical gauge for who should get what treatment. Women would be faced with far fewer difficult choices if we could finely calibrate the risks and the treatments and come up each time with a precise plan of what to do. You would then get pretty much the same advice from every doctor you spoke to.

Unfortunately, the treatments now available to us do not permit such fine tuning. What is considered "aggressive treatment" very much depends on whom you are talking to. The routine approach of one doctor may be considered aggressive by another.

There are, however, a few criteria by which such judgments are commonly made:

- CMF is considered the standard treatment for most women with node-positive breast cancer.
- If the oncologist were to propose using only MF, that would be considered less aggressive treatment.
- If she used a combination like CAF, FAC, or CMFVP, certain other physicians might consider that more aggressive.
- Alternating drug combinations, the intensity of dosage, and the intervals between treatments are other variables used to differentiate how vigorous the treatment is.

What are the opinions you are likely to be given for your particular circumstance? The following chart may help explain what treatment an oncologist may recommend for you. (Refer to earlier sections of this chapter for explanations of the drug combinations that follow, as well as the various rationales for their use.)

```
                         − Nodes +
Group        1  2    3    4       5          6
Lower risk —+——+——+——|——————————+———— Higher risk
```

Group 1 = Microinvasion, no involved nodes

Group 2 = Tumor less than 1 cm, no involved nodes

Group 3 = Tumor more than 1 cm, no involved nodes

Group 4 = 1–3 involved nodes

Group 5 = 4–9 nodes

Group 6 = 10 or more nodes

Premenopausal Women

If you are in Groups One and Two:

- No treatment may be recommended because of your relatively low risk.
- A "less aggressive" treatment like MF with leucovorin may be suggested.
- CMF or less toxic variations of CMFVP may be used by some oncologists.

If you are in Group Three, chemotherapy is desirable and one of the following drug combinations may be suggested:

- MF/leucovorin
- CMF
- CMFVP
- CAF

If you are in Group Four, one of the following treatments will be proposed:

- CMF
- CMFVP
- CAF and its variants

If you are in Group Five, one of the following treatments will be proposed:

- CAF and its variants
- Adria/CMF and its variants
- Sequential high-dose regimens
- Very-high-dose chemotherapy with bone-marrow and/or stem-cell transplant

Group Six patients will be presented with the greatest range of options. CMF alone is not effective, but each of the following programs offers some promise of helping. Most oncologists have developed regimens for this group that they feel provide optimal responses. You will undoubtedly be offered one of the following:

- CAF
- FAC
- Adria/CMF and its variants
- Sequential high-dose regimens
- Very-high-dose regimens with bone-marrow and/or stem-cell transplant

Postmenopausal Women

Most oncologists prescribe tamoxifen for women in all groups who have positive hormone receptors. The drug's usefulness, as we have discussed, is less clear for women who are hormone-receptor negative.

If you are hormone-receptor positive and in Group One or Two, one of the following may be suggested:

- No treatment because of the relatively low risk
- Tamoxifen only
- Tamoxifen plus a "less aggressive" treatment like MF with leucovorin

If you are in Group Three, with negative nodes and a tumor that was larger than one centimeter, you may be offered one of the following:

- Tamoxifen only
- Tamoxifen plus MF/leucovorin
- Tamoxifen plus CMF
- Tamoxifen plus CMFVP

If you are in Group Four, with fewer than three positive nodes, you may be offered one of the following:

- Tamoxifen only
- Tamoxifen plus CMFVP
- Tamoxifen plus CAF or its variants

If you are in Group Five, with four to nine involved nodes, you may be offered one of the following:

- Tamoxifen only
- Tamoxifen plus CAF
- Tamoxifen plus FAC
- Tamoxifen plus Adria/CMF and its variants
- Sequential high-dosage regimens

If you are in Group Six, with ten or more involved nodes, you may be offered one of the following:

- CAF
- FAC
- Adria/CMF and its variants
- Sequential high-dosage regimens
- Very-high-dosage regimens with bone-marrow and/or stem-cell transplant

For women who are postmenopausal and hormone-receptor negative, chemotherapy can also be of value. Some oncologists may use tamoxifen in addition to chemotherapy.

For Group One, no treatment may be used because of the relatively low risk.

For Groups Two and Three on the chart—women with no node involvement—one of the following may be used:

- MF/leucovorin
- CMF
- CMFVP

For Group Four, CMF is not of any value and the following options may be suggested:

- CMFVP
- CAF and its variants

If you are in Group Five the following options may be suggested:

- CAF
- FAC

- Adria/CMF
- Sequential high-dosage regimens
- Very-high-dosage regimens with bone-marrow and/or stem-cell transplant

For Group Six, suggested treatments may include the following:

- CAF
- FAC
- Adria/CMF and its variants
- Sequential high-dosage regimens
- Very-high-dosage regimens with bone-marrow and/or stem-cell transplant

Chemotherapy to Reduce Tumor Size Before Surgery

Chemotherapy (or neo-adjuvant chemotherapy, as it is called in this context) is sometimes used to treat very large tumors before surgery. The programs commonly used for this purpose are CAF or CMFVP.

IN SUMMARY

I recommend preventive hormone therapy or chemotherapy to all patients with invasive cancers because it seems to me that even a small risk of a life-threatening recurrence of breast cancer is unacceptable if there is a chance that risk can be reduced. There are situations, as with very small invasive tumors, where it is very hard to ask a woman to go through a course of treatment she probably dreads and that may have some temporary side effects. But even in these instances, it seems clearly better to do everything we can to prevent a recurrence of cancer.

The development of preventive therapy has changed the prospects of tens of thousands of women. It has also given us hope that someday, with improved therapy, all women will be cured of breast cancer.

11

BREAST
RECONSTRUCTION

❧❧❧

R eplacing the breast after mastectomy by means of breast reconstruction is elective surgery. That means there is no compelling medical reason for the operation. Whether or not you choose to have this procedure is entirely your call. The choice became more complicated in 1992, however, when the Food and Drug Administration ordered that the use of silicone-gel implants for cosmetic purposes be discontinued because certain manufacturers may not have been forthcoming about the potential risks of using these implants. Several scientific studies have subsequently proven the safety of silicone implants. Nevertheless, as a result of major ongoing suits alleging damage, several manufacturers went out of business. The use of silicone-filled implants is now reserved only for breast reconstruction after mastectomy, and then under "limited supervisory" conditions. Realistically, they are not available and have been replaced by saline-filled implants. This matter is discussed more fully later in this chapter.

We know that women have very different reactions to the removal of their breasts. There are also a variety of reasons why some do not want breast reconstruction:

- They seem relatively undisturbed about losing a breast, glad to be alive without worrying too much about the cosmetic effects of mastectomy.

- They do not want to have more general anesthesia or to undergo further surgery.

- Especially if they were small-breasted to begin with, there may not be enough real difference in their appearance when they are dressed to bother them.

- They are satisfied with their appearance when they are dressed and wearing a prosthesis (see page 193) inside their bra.

- They feel that it is a betrayal of what they have lived through to hide the fact that they had breast surgery in order to conform to society's definition of what a woman's body should look like.

- They are concerned about the recent questions that have been raised about the safety of silicone-gel implants.

On the other hand, there are many, many women who, after mastectomy, feel that having both breasts is vital to their physical and emotional health. For them, what is at stake is their own self-image and their sense of the wholeness of their bodies.

It is this same feeling, of course (and its effectiveness), that has made the lumpectomy procedure as common as it is today. But the truth is that the choice between mastectomy and lumpectomy no longer needs to make such a radical difference cosmetically. The techniques of breast reconstruction have become so refined that though they might still prefer to have been able to preserve their breasts, women who have had mastectomies and reconstruction also feel good about their appearance. And if the reconstruction is done at the time of the mastectomy, even the trauma of waking up after surgery with one side of the body totally different from the other can be avoided.

THE CHOICES

Do Nothing

You can choose to do nothing cosmetically after mastectomy, as women regularly did in the past and many continue to do now. What are the consequences? They vary.

I asked one of my patients who had been quite vehement about not having reconstruction what she thought about her decision six months after her surgery. She said hastily, "I'm fine, I'm fine. I'm just careful when I get dressed in the morning not to look in the mirror. I never look in the mirror when I'm undressed."

It seems to me this woman is not as "fine" as she said she was. On the other hand, another patient—a particularly chic professional woman—seems genuinely accepting of a double mastectomy. She now wears clothes that are cut differently from those she wore before the surgery, but finds that no great hardship. She has been married for a long time and says that her husband has grown more appreciative of her since the cancer than he was before.

The conclusion about doing nothing? Many women seem to fare well, others less well.

Wear a Prosthesis

You can decline to have reconstruction and, instead, consider wearing a prosthesis, an artificial breast form.

1. Can I try a prosthesis before actually buying one?

There is an easy way to accomplish this. Usually, after you have had a mastectomy, a volunteer from the American Cancer Society's Reach to Recovery program (see page 125) or someone from the hospital breast service will visit you in the hospital. This person will provide you with a bra that contains a temporary cloth prosthesis and will encourage you to wear it home from the hospital and during the following weeks. It won't fit as well as a permanent prosthesis, but it will give you the idea of how your clothes will look with the prosthesis in place.

2. What is a permanent prosthesis like?

The prosthesis is often a plastic form that contains silicone gel and is therefore fairly resilient and soft to the touch. Another type is made from nylon and cotton and is cushioned with a fiber mixed with tiny glass beads that are said to give the form weight and balance.

3. When will I be ready to use one?

You can be fitted for a permanent prosthesis within two to three weeks after your surgery, when there is no longer any swelling and your surgeon says the wound no longer needs care.

4. Where do I get a good prosthesis?

The local unit of the American Cancer Society, or a Reach to Recovery volunteer, or the nurse in your surgeon's office will be able to give you a list of vendors.

Corset shops and the lingerie departments of many large department stores employ salespeople with special experience in working with women who have had mastectomies.

There are also shops that specialize in postmastectomy fittings. These usually stock a variety of forms and will also sew pockets in your own bras to accommodate the prosthesis.

Try to find out before you go there whether other people have been satisfied with the work of the store you're considering. A good fitter is important. If you are small-breasted, it may only be necessary to use some light padding. If you are fairly heavy-breasted, the weight will have to be evenly balanced so that your bra does not ride up on one side, and so that you avoid back and shoulder strain.

5. What will it look like when I'm wearing one?

The results, when you are dressed or wearing a bra, are so good that you will look the same as you always have. The variety of prosthesis shapes and sizes enables you to come fairly close to matching the shape and weight of your own breast.

Reconstruction

Though many women are satisfied to wear a prosthesis, others are not:

- "Every time I put it into my bra, I remember that I had breast cancer."

194

- "Even with the form, I feel unbalanced."
- "When I'd go out for my run in the morning, especially in the summer, I'd always be worrying that the prosthesis was going to pop out."
- "A prosthesis isn't the point. I'm not worried about what other people think about the way I look, I'm the one I care about. I don't like the feeling that I'm missing a vital part, especially one that's been so important to my life. I don't only mean my sex life—I mean things like nursing my babies, and looking in the mirror and admiring my great shape."

More and more women are choosing breast reconstruction after mastectomy. According to the American Society of Plastic and Reconstructive Surgeons, in 1994 over 26,000 women had breast reconstruction, and today's figures are almost certainly higher.

For about 16,000 of those women an implant or expander was used; for about 9,000 it was their own body tissue that was employed to reconstruct the breast. Though the latter procedure continues to be less common, there is reason to believe that in coming years more women will choose it.

WHO DOES BREAST RECONSTRUCTION?

You should go to a reconstructive surgeon, a plastic surgeon who regularly does breast reconstruction. A plastic surgeon who sees mostly postaccident patients or primarily does cosmetic procedures probably does not have sufficient current experience in breast reconstruction. As in the search for other specialists, the governing philosophy is that the more of this procedure the surgeon does, the better.

He should be board-certified, with special training and experience in plastic surgery and breast reconstruction, having passed an examination in the specialty.

Almost certainly, the best referral you can get is from your breast surgeon. For one thing, it's important to him that you be satisfied with the combined results of mastectomy and reconstruction. There will be one or two people with whom he has worked and whose results he respects.

In addition, discuss with other women who have had reconstruction which plastic surgeons they used and whether they were satisfied with the results. For specific advice on finding a doctor, refer to Chapter Two.

Talk at length to one or two plastic surgeons before making your final decision to make sure that your goals for the procedure and those of the person you choose coincide. For example, if you are quite small-breasted, some plastic surgeons may recommend that, for what are to them aesthetic reasons, the second breast also be augmented. Don't have surgery merely to conform to someone else's idea of what is cosmetically pleasing. If you've always wanted larger breasts, this may be the time to achieve that goal, but that should be exclusively your own judgment. (On the other hand, if you are especially full-breasted, it may not be possible to make your reconstructed breast as large as the remaining one and the second breast is frequently reduced.)

THE COST OF RECONSTRUCTION

The cost varies according to the type of procedure and where in the country you're having it. For reasons that will become clear as we discuss each procedure, the simple insertion of an implant costs less than a free-flap reconstruction. The creation of a nipple raises the cost of all reconstruction.

As one example of what these procedures cost, in New York City, flap surgery can add seven to sixteen thousand dollars to the cost of a mastectomy.

Reconstruction after mastectomy is not considered cosmetic surgery, as many people believe. Most insurance companies, therefore, pay for a reconstruction; but whether they will pay for the more expensive procedures varies from policy to policy. Check with your benefits representative or with the insurer. Talk to someone at the local division of the American Cancer Society and to your breast surgeon, as well as the plastic surgeon, about finding help to pay for reconstruction.

WHEN IS RECONSTRUCTION DONE?

Because it used to be thought that breast implants at the site of mastectomies might mask the recurrence of cancer or even cause it, reconstruction was delayed until it was considered "safe," usually at least five years after mastectomy. Most of the time the procedure is now done at the time of the mastectomy, as soon as the breast surgeon has finished his work. That means that the plastic surgeon must practice at the same hospital as the breast surgeon and must be available at the time of the operation. This can limit the choice of plastic surgeons, though the scheduling conflicts can usually be overcome.

Years of experience have shown that breast reconstruction after mastectomy does not appear to interfere with any post-surgical treatment you may need. Nor does it mask or interfere with the detection of cancer or increase its risk *after a mastectomy has been performed.*

Mammographies are not performed on a reconstructed breast, but when a mammogram is taken of an intact breast in which an implant has been inserted for augmentation, it is more difficult to get a clear visualization of the breast tissue. Additional X-ray views are required.

Now that lumpectomy is so prevalent a form of treatment, women who had counted on preserving their breast are sometimes very disheartened if they are advised that this procedure is not appropriate for their particular condition. When immediate breast reconstruction is an option, it can make the prospect of mastectomy much less traumatic.

Other women prefer to wait until they've recovered from their surgery, had a chance to catch their breath, think about it at leisure, and talk it over with family and friends. There are a great many important decisions to make and much to absorb emotionally and physically in the weeks after breast cancer is diagnosed, so it is not at all uncommon to feel you need time before you make another decision.

In such instances, where the reconstruction is not done at the time of the mastectomy, most surgeons recommend that you allow a three-month period for the mastectomy site to heal. Breast reconstruction is feasible any time after that—even years later. It is really never too late.

The Implant

An implant is really an internal prosthesis, a plastic envelope filled with a saline solution or with silicone gel or with a combination of these.

The implant is not placed, as many people think, directly under the skin. Instead, it is inserted under the chest muscle, in a pocket created by the surgeon. The muscle lies over the implant, girdling it.

Implants are inserted in a surgical procedure, usually under general anesthesia.

If the implant is not done at the time of the mastectomy, a small incision will be made in the skin, usually at the side or in the crease at the base of the breast site.

Breast implant placement

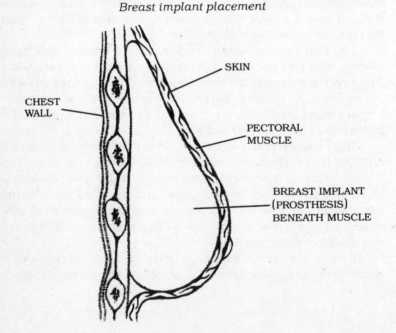

CHEST WALL

SKIN

PECTORAL MUSCLE

BREAST IMPLANT (PROSTHESIS) BENEATH MUSCLE

A drain is inserted to remove any fluids that accumulate in the days after surgery. This is later removed.

The incision is closed with sutures, as in any surgery.

Implant surgery takes about one and a half hours.

In addition to these standard elements of all breast implants, there are variations in the procedures:

In a simple implant, the full-sized implant can be put in place in one operation, especially if the skin is sturdy and can be stretched, the chest muscle is healthy, and the woman is small- or average-breasted.

Much more common in the past several years is a procedure called tissue expansion. A small balloonlike device is placed under the chest muscle. It contains a valve into which saline solution can be injected.

About once a week, for an average of eight to ten weeks, additional saline solution is injected through the skin and into the balloon. As the device expands, the skin and the muscles slowly stretch and grow until the right size is achieved. The process is exactly like what happens when your breasts and abdomen stretch to accommodate a pregnancy.

Tissue expansion

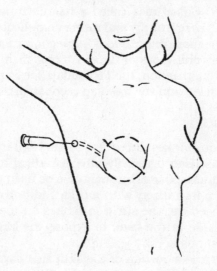

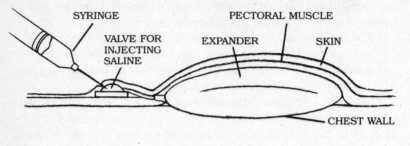

Tissue expander

Saline is added to the expander until it has reached a size somewhat larger than the planned permanent implant, in order that the stretched skin will create a more natural appearance once the procedure is completed. The expander is then removed, usually under general anesthesia, and the permanent implant is put in place.

Reconstruction with Your Own Tissue

Breast reconstruction can be accomplished using your own skin, muscle, and fat. Sometimes called a tissue transfer or a myocutaneous flap, these lengthy and rather complicated procedures can result in the most natural-looking reconstructions.

There are several types of flaps. Among them are the latissimus dorsi reconstruction; the TRAM flap (for transverse rectus abdominal muscle); and the free flap reconstruction.

LATISSIMUS DORSI

This procedure takes about five to six hours under general anesthesia. It is used primarily after a radical mastectomy to replace the pectoral muscle, but may also be used to reconstruct a small breast in its entirety without the addition of an implant. During the procedure, the surgeon makes an incision beneath the shoulder blade in the back to expose the large flat muscle called the latissimus dorsi.

The muscle and a portion of the skin that covers it are then moved, through a tunnel created under the skin, from the pa-

200

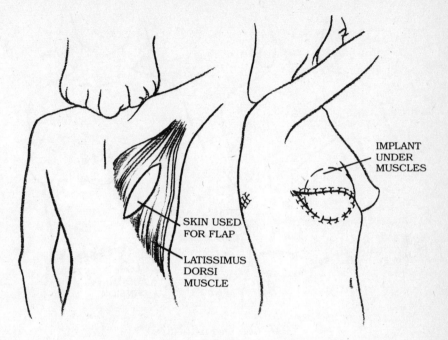

IMPLANT
UNDER
MUSCLES

SKIN USED
FOR FLAP

LATISSIMUS
DORSI
MUSCLE

Latissimus dorsi flap reconstruction

tient's back to the site of the mastectomy. An implant is usually needed, and is placed under the latissimus dorsi muscle now relocated at the mastectomy site. Drains are inserted to remove any fluid that may accumulate over the following few days, and sutures are used to close the incision. (See Chapter Seven if you wish to review general procedures for breast surgery.)

Obviously, because the skin just under the shoulder blade is being cut, there will be a scar on the back as well as on the chest.

TRAM FLAP

This procedure can take five to eight hours under general anesthesia and can result in a quite natural reconstruction. The newly constructed breast will respond to changes in weight just as the rest of the body does. The TRAM flap is not suitable for women who are very thin or extremely obese, who have abdominal scars from previous surgery, or who are heavy smokers.

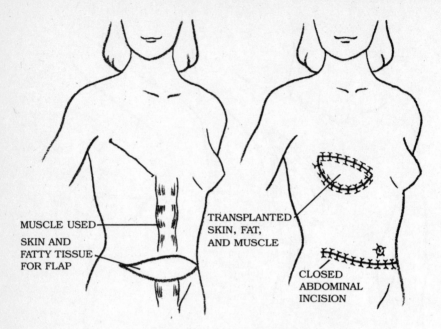

MUSCLE USED

SKIN AND
FATTY TISSUE
FOR FLAP

TRANSPLANTED
SKIN, FAT,
AND MUSCLE

CLOSED
ABDOMINAL
INCISION

TRAM flap reconstruction

Occasionally, before the actual surgery, a preliminary procedure called a delay is performed in which a blood vessel is tied off to improve the circulation to the tissue of the flap. During the TRAM flap procedure, your own tissue is moved, still connected to its blood supply (called a pedicle), from one part of the body to another. If the blood vessels are retained, it is called a pedicle flap; if cut, it is called a free flap. The surgeon makes an elliptical incision in the lower abdomen. He then moves the skin, the fat, the blood vessels, and one or both of the abdominal muscles, through a tunnel he creates under the skin, from the abdomen to the mastectomy site.

This flap of muscle, skin, and fat is contoured into the shape of your breast. Usually there is enough fat so that an implant is not required. The procedure does, of course, leave a large scar across the abdomen. The results of the abdominal surgery are very much like those of a cosmetic procedure called an abdominal plasty or "tummy tuck."

Drains will be placed in the incisions to remove the fluid that collects over the next few days. Both incisions will be closed with sutures.

FREE FLAP RECONSTRUCTION

This procedure takes six to twelve hours under general anesthetic and requires the services of a plastic surgeon who is skilled in microsurgery, a technique that makes it possible to sew together hair-thin blood vessels so that normal blood flow can take place.

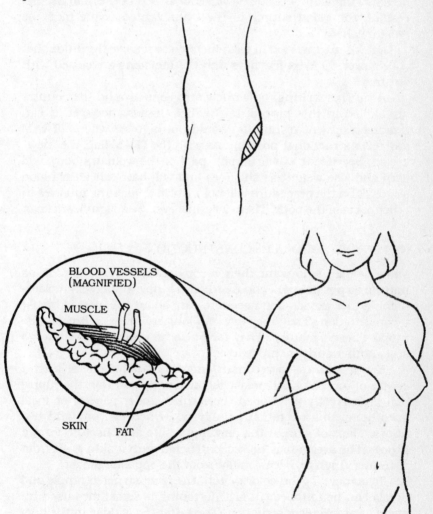

BLOOD VESSELS
(MAGNIFIED)

MUSCLE

SKIN   FAT

Free flap reconstruction

Instead of preserving the blood supply, as in the standard pedicle TRAM reconstruction, a wedge of tissue is cut out of the buttock or thigh. It is as if you were amputating this tissue, with its vein and artery, and then reattaching it at the site of the mastectomy. There the artery and vein are reconnected, this time to the blood vessels that formerly nourished the region of the breast. This is important, because for this procedure to be successful, the blood supply to the transplanted tissue must be reestablished.

Drains are inserted in each incision to remove the fluids that collect over the next few days and the incisions are closed with sutures.

As of this writing, only a few surgeons around the country are skilled in this procedure. In their hands, however, it can produce excellent results. It should not be used when a TRAM flap reconstruction is possible. As with the TRAM flap, the "new" breast, because it was originally part of the woman's body, will gain and lose weight as she does and will have a healthy blood supply; and the procedure will not involve weakening muscles in other parts of the body. There will, however, be a significant scar.

NIPPLE AND AREOLA RECONSTRUCTION

Many women who want their reconstructed breast to look as natural as possible will choose to have nipple and areola replacement. Other women don't seem to care about this part of breast reconstruction. They may say, "As long as I have a breast, the nipple doesn't matter." They may also be reluctant to undergo still another surgical procedure.

Nipple and areola reconstruction is usually done at least a couple of months after breast reconstruction so that the nipple can be correctly positioned. Performed under general or local anesthetic, this operation usually takes between one and two hours. Flaps of skin at the new nipple site are raised to form a nipple. The areola may be reconstructed with a skin graft from the inner thigh or, occasionally, from the opposite breast.

To achieve a good color match, the reconstructed nipple and areola can be tattooed; in fact, tattooing is sometimes used instead of nipple reconstruction. The tattooing is done in the doctor's office, under local anesthetic.

Side Effects of Breast Reconstruction

PAIN?

There is, of course, some pain associated with all surgery, since it involves the cutting and manipulation of tissue. There is relatively little pain as a result of mastectomy. Breast implants, however, do cause more temporary discomfort because of the pressure of the prosthesis against the chest wall as well as the stretching of the muscle.

Where tissue is moved from one part of the body to another, there will be two wounds that may cause you discomfort, and with the TRAM flap you will have the greater discomfort that is associated with abdominal surgery. Some numbness will remain in the lower central abdomen after a TRAM flap, and there will be widening of the hips in short-waisted women.

During a TRAM flap, a hernia, or hole, may develop in the fascia, the fibrous tissue that gives the abdominal wall its strength. This is a rare occurrence, but these hernias eventually have to be repaired.

Since tissue transfers may involve considerable blood loss, you may need a transfusion. Prepare for this in advance of the surgery by donating your own blood or having friends and family do so. This blood will be stored specifically for your use, in case you need it.

HARDENING OF THE BREAST

When there has been an implant, it is expected that scar tissue will form around it, as the body works to encapsulate this "foreign" insertion. The extent of the scarring depends on the woman's own physiology. Sometimes, this *capsular contracture*, as it is called, may become quite hard, and it can sometimes be painful.

If this happens, the incision may be opened by the plastic surgeon, some of the scarring surgically "broken up," and a new implant inserted. This is not commonly done after breast reconstruction.

RIPPLING OF THE IMPLANT SURFACE

Saline implants that are underfilled may have a "wavy" appearance and feel soft to the touch. Others that are overfilled may be too firm. The plastic surgeon will try to find a happy medium.

WEAKENING OF THE ABDOMINAL MUSCLES

Because the TRAM flap (see above) involves an incision and transfer of muscle from the abdominal region, stomach tone may be lost. (On the other hand, since fat is removed, it may also make your stomach look better because, as we have noted, the procedure actually does result in a tummy tuck.)

TISSUE FAILURE

The major complication of flap reconstruction is the occasional failure of the transferred tissue to survive. If this happens, part or all of the tissue will have to be removed and the wound may require an extended period of treatment and revision by the surgeon before it heals.

INFECTION

Infections may develop at the site of any surgery in the period just after the procedure. They are treated with antibiotics and generally respond well. During an infection, an implant may have to be temporarily removed. Most often it can be reinserted several months after the infection is gone.

LEAKAGE

When a saline solution is used, there may be some leakage from the prosthesis. Leakage of this type poses no danger since the "salt water" is simply absorbed into the body tissues. The implant, however, will deflate and have to be replaced.

It is leakage from silicone gel-filled implants that is the cause of the recent concern and the recent actions of the Food and Drug Administration. There have been reports that silicone-gel leakage may be associated with serious autoimmune diseases, such as scleroderma and arthritis. The American College of Rheumatology stated in late 1995 that there is no evidence of a causal relationship between silicone-gel exposure and any of the rheumatoid diseases. Furthermore, as we have noted, a number of scientific studies have confirmed the safety of these implants.

These studies were reported *after* the FDA banned their use for cosmetic purposes and imposed "supervisory" conditions over their use for breast reconstruction after mastectomy. However, much damage has been done by the class action lawsuits against the manufacturers that it is unlikely silicone-gel implants will be available for years to come, if ever.

Implants have been used for over thirty years, primarily— over eighty percent—for cosmetic, not reconstruction purposes. None of the recent data have made the distinction between the two uses, so we don't know precisely what percentage of postmastectomy patients have had difficulty with silicone-gel implants.

As we have seen, saline solution is always used in the expansion step of the reconstruction process. At this time we really have no alternative to using saline-filled permanent implants as well. Research is under way to find substitutes.

DETERIORATION OF THE PROSTHESIS

Polyurethane has sometimes been used to cover implants in order to avoid hardening of the tissue around them. Reports of animal experiments seem to indicate that the polyurethane coating in the **Même** and **Replicon** brand inserts has deteriorated. Because the breakdown products of polyurethane may be carcinogenic, further study is now under way and the manufacturer has withdrawn these products from the market. No carcinogenic effect has ever been demonstrated in humans.

If you have had an implant, you should speak to your plastic surgeon and find out whether a polyurethane-covered device was used. As of this writing, however, there is certainly not enough information available to warrant the removal of such implants. In fact, the risk of cancer from a polyurethane implant is thought to be far less than the risk associated with the implant's removal. Follow news reports on this subject carefully and stay in touch with your plastic surgeon.

Most medical procedures have side effects. As we saw when we talked about mastectomy and lumpectomy, there are factors to be weighed, risks and benefits to be balanced.

As of this writing, the Food and Drug Administration has ordered that manufacturers stop distributing silicone gel-filled implants and that physicians stop inserting them for cosmetic purposes. Dr. David A. Kessler, the commissioner of the FDA, has said that women who are not experiencing problems need not consider having implants removed, but that those who are having symptoms they think may be related to the implants should see their doctors. In fact, all women with implants should have regular examinations by their surgeons.

You do not have to have reconstructive surgery right after mastectomy. Many women will probably opt to wait until the present situation has been clarified. If, however, you do want to have the procedure immediately, discuss with the surgeon the use of a saline-filled implant.

We have to learn a lot more about these matters as soon as possible, using as much meticulous care as possible. If there is a problem with the present implants we should find safe substitutes for postmastectomy patients to whom breast reconstruction is important. There is little doubt that reconstruction procedures have made an enormous difference in the overall well-being of most patients who have used them. Breast reconstruction after mastectomy has enhanced the lives of many women by enabling them to live their lives with a feeling of wholeness, and with no apparent sacrifice of their physical well-being.

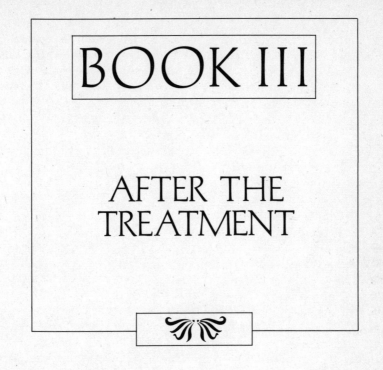

BOOK III

AFTER THE TREATMENT

CHAPTER

12

FOLLOW-UP

❧

Near the beginning of the book, to show how complex the experience of breast cancer can be, we used as a contrast the example of appendicitis, with its straightforward protocol of treatment. Dealing with breast cancer is complicated not only because of all the treatment options, but also because of what is required after the disease has been treated.

After an appendectomy, when the stitches have been removed and you have regained your strength, you can say goodbye to your surgeon and not concern yourself with the illness anymore. It's over.

After breast cancer, to take care of yourself properly involves a lifetime of surveillance. That doesn't mean you're going to be in a state of high anxiety all the time, or that you will have to go for frequent and expensive tests and examinations for the rest of your life. But it does mean careful follow-up and monitoring of your condition, especially for the first three or four years after your surgery.

WHY THE FOLLOW-UP?

Because breast cancer has a tendency to recur locally and also to spread to other parts of the body, in addition to your surgery, you are likely to have received radiation and perhaps hormone therapy and/or chemotherapy unless you had a tiny or non-invasive cancer.

The purpose of careful follow-up is to detect any recurrence, either local or systemic, at the earliest possible time, so it can be treated most effectively. (Recurrence will be discussed in Chapter Thirteen.)

After Mastectomy

Even if you had a mastectomy, there is the possibility that you may have a local recurrence of breast cancer in the area where the breast used to be, most commonly at the site of the mastectomy incision on the chest wall. Microscopic cancer cells may have been lurking in adjacent tissue. Such cells can remain undetected for an indeterminate time—perhaps a few months, perhaps many years.

Cancer may also recur in the lymph nodes in the axilla and the neck. This is called a regional recurrence. Distant recurrence is used to describe the finding of cancer that has spread to other parts of the body.

After Lumpectomy

Even following radiation therapy after a lumpectomy, there is a certain risk that microscopic cancer remains in the tissue adjacent to the site of the original cancer. Therefore, in the first few years after lumpectomy, the most common place for the cancer to recur is, in fact, in the area of the original tumor site.

A recurrence in the breast is less worrisome than other recurrences because it does not indicate that the original cancer has metastasized. There is an excellent chance that with further surgery and adjuvant therapy, we can eliminate the problem.

A new cancer can also develop elsewhere in the breast, just as a new cancer can develop in the opposite breast. Such new and separate breast cancers—as well as regional and systemic cancers—do remain a risk over a woman's lifetime in the sense that the risk factors that played a part in the first cancer may still be present.

WHO'S IN CHARGE OF THE FOLLOW-UP?

As we have emphasized throughout the book, in an important sense you are the one in charge. In this instance, it is up to you to make sure that no one says to you after surgery and any adjuvant treatment, "Okay, you're fine. Case dismissed." It is also important that you yourself don't say, "Okay, it's over. Good-bye. Leave me alone."

Neither you nor your doctors can resign. Stay alert yourself and put into place a team that will take the "necessary precautions":

1. Make sure there is a follow-up plan in place. (See below.)

2. Decide which doctor is going to be in charge. This question was important during the treatment of your breast cancer and now comes up again. You are not in any way obligated to remain with the last person to treat your breast cancer for the follow-up. You can give the matter some thought, and if you decide to make a change, choose who, among the specialists who have been treating you, would do the best job.

3. The surgeon was the leader of the team before, during, and after the operation, and he may be the best person to act as coordinator in the years that follow, to help evaluate or interpret the various options that may arise. This is

213

especially true if further surgery is indicated. A surgeon, whether the original one or someone you now choose, should also do ongoing examinations of your breasts after lumpectomy, or of the one remaining breast.

4. If you need long-term hormone therapy or chemotherapy, or if further surgery is not planned, it may be that your oncologist will be the doctor you select to stay in charge of your case.

5. Some women want their follow-up to be supervised by their own family physician, usually an internist, especially if they have had a good long-term relationship with her. That doctor should certainly be kept informed, and she can help you judge how your treatment is progressing, but it is almost certain that you will be better off being monitored by a cancer specialist. In this regard, the specialist will serve as a consultant to the doctor who is responsible for other aspects of your health.

6. Though who becomes the head of your team may come about naturally and satisfactorily, you may want to speak directly to the physician you consider the most caring, meticulous, and alert, and specifically ask her to stay on top of your case.

7. In addition to treating you, the person you choose as the "main woman" or "main man" must maintain careful records of all the tests and treatments you will receive, of the state of your health in terms of cancer as well as of your general medical condition, and—it seems to me— of how your whole life is going.

THE FOLLOW-UP SCHEDULE

There is no standard "calendar of events" that plots how often you should see each physician in the years ahead. The frequency depends to a large degree on the extent of the illness at the time of diagnosis, and also on how much time has passed since your treatment.

Unless you had a mastectomy without any other therapy or reconstruction, it's likely that you'll be seeing some combination of surgeon, chemotherapist, radiotherapist, or plastic surgeon on and off for at least six months, and probably for the first year, after your surgery.

After this period of intensive treatment, for the first three or four years you should see the surgeon every six months.

If you had a lumpectomy followed by radiation therapy, ideally you should alternate the visits to the surgeon with visits to the radiation therapist every six months.

If you are receiving long-term chemotherapy, the oncologist, as you have seen, will also be examining you on a regular basis and conducting tests.

It is because you will be visiting several different specialists that you need someone at the center of your care to keep track of what each physician is doing and finding.

WHAT DOES FOLLOW-UP INVOLVE?

Physical Examination

Every six months you should have a complete physical examination, from head to toe. If you are seeing an oncologist, it is usually she who will perform this examination. Otherwise an internist familiar with your case should examine you.

If a mastectomy was performed, this doctor will physically examine the chest wall as well as the lymph nodes in the region of the armpit and neck. He will also carefully examine the remaining breast.

If there was a lumpectomy, the treated breast will be carefully palpated to see whether there is any suspicion of a new lump, and the other breast also will be examined.

Tests

In order for us to achieve fairly uniform reporting of results, many of the same tests are used for all patients. In addition, specific tests are tailored to each patient's circumstance. (The most common exceptions arise when a patient is enrolled in a clinical study. In that case, her follow-up is governed by the rules of the study. Such studies are discussed in Chapter Fifteen.) It is important to say from the start, though, that no single test can ever be relied upon for a definitive diagnosis of breast cancer.

BLOOD TESTS

A complete blood count should be done every six months. It tells us a number of things: the total number and size of red blood cells; the total volume of the red cells in proportion to the total volume of blood (called the hematocrit); and the hemoglobin content—that is, the quantity in the blood of the protein that carries oxygen.

The blood count also measures the number of circulating white blood cells and of platelets, the cell particles in the blood involved in forming clots.

A mildly reduced hematocrit or hemoglobin may be a sign of chronic illness or of diabetes, arthritis, or heavy menstrual bleeding. If the hematocrit or hemoglobin is very low, anemia is present, and we would have to be concerned about the possibility that this is due to tumor recurrence. The same would be true if there were a very low white cell or platelet count.

Blood chemistries, another type of blood test, measure various chemicals in the bloodstream. One enzyme that is of special interest in breast cancer is alkaline phosphatase. When it is present in elevated amounts, we are concerned about recurrence in either bone or liver, though there are other possible causes of this elevation. Other chemistries raise concern about liver involvement specifically.

Blood tests called tumor marker tests usually show abnormal results only when a tumor is large enough to release detectable quantities of certain substances. These tests therefore alert us to the presence of tumors of significant size.

CEA (carcino-embryonic antigen), one such marker, is released in normal amounts by glandular tissue, but in increased amounts by tumor cells. Increased production of a milk-fat globule protein, CA15-3, another marker, is a more sensitive test for breast cancer. Because this test is not yet approved by the FDA, it is considered experimental and you may find that your insurance will not cover the cost. A test similar to CA15-3 is BR 27/29.

Blood cholesterol and lipid metabolism measurements are also useful in monitoring general health.

MAMMOGRAPHY

Every woman who has had breast cancer should have a mammogram once a year. If she has had a single mastectomy, the remaining breast should be X-rayed. If she has had a lumpectomy, both breasts should be X-rayed. A reconstructed breast is not X-rayed.

CHEST X RAYS

A chest X ray will tell us whether any cancer has spread to the lung, a common site of metastasis. You should have a chest X ray every year, and if you have a cough or shortness of breath, more frequent X rays may be necessary.

BONE SCANS

If the initial cancer was invasive, a bone scan (a special study of the bones) is done to see whether there is any involvement of the bones and also to establish a baseline, a measurement we can use to judge future conditions. There is some difference of opinion about how often bone scans should be used. Some oncologists insist on a scan at regular intervals, but others of us feel that it should not be used routinely. There is, however, no question that a bone scan is necessary if there are symptoms such as persistent back, joint, or other bone pain. Since these symptoms are worrisome, only a negative bone scan can provide peace of mind.

To prepare for a bone scan, a radioactive liquid is injected into the bloodstream and allowed to circulate throughout the body. The liquid will go to the bones and reveal the skeletal system. It will concentrate in areas of increased blood circulation, referred to as hot spots. These include areas of arthritis or bone fractures, as well as those where cancer is present.

For that reason, though a bone scan is a very sensitive tool for finding bone metastases, its results have to be confirmed with X rays to identify more precisely the reason the scan has shown increased blood circulation in any particular bone.

OTHER TESTS

The tests we have discussed are the ones routinely used in follow-up care to guard against a recurrence of breast cancer. If blood tests suggest that there may be an abnormality of the liver, the most practical tool to investigate this is a CAT scan (see page 69)

217

of the abdomen. Sonography (see page 68) and MRI (see page 69) may also be used for further study. Other tests are used only when unusual questions arise.

FOR HOW LONG WILL I NEED THESE TESTS?

We talked earlier in the book about five-year survival rates. While there's nothing magical about that anniversary, the fact is that most local recurrences, as well as metastases, occur in the first two or three years after surgery. (Sometimes, when the breast was treated with lumpectomy and radiation, there can be later local recurrences.)

But for women with early disease, if there has been no recurrence in five years, it's quite all right to relax. You need your annual physical examination, blood tests, chest X ray, and mammogram, but you don't need to be examined any more often than that.

Women with more advanced disease will probably see the oncologist over a longer period of time and will therefore have more frequent follow-up examinations. They will also be closely watched by the surgeon for a longer time. For these women, the switch can be made to annual examinations after ten disease-free years.

Watching Out for Yourself

In addition to the professional tests and examinations, you should continue breast self-examination. Some women say that they're reluctant to start examining themselves again after breast surgery, either because they dread finding another cancer or because they're a little squeamish about touching their treated breast or the chest wall after a mastectomy. This feeling seems to pass after a few months.

Even if you share these reactions, do not neglect your self-examination:

- Examine your breasts and the operative area carefully every month.
- If you have had a breast reconstruction, ask the plastic surgeon to show you how to examine your treated breast.

He should point out to you the location of any valve or other protuberance in an implant so that you don't mistake it for a lump.

- Whether you had a lumpectomy or a mastectomy, ask the surgeon to show you how to examine the scar. First, notice whether there is a rash over the incision. Then, carefully move the pads of your fingers up and then down the skin over the scar, palpating in the same way discussed on page 52.

- If you had a mastectomy, you are watching for a lump on the chest wall, beneath the skin, frequently beneath the scar.

- If you had a lumpectomy, you are watching for a lump or change in breast consistency in the treated breast.

- A lump in the neck or under the arm may indicate an enlarged lymph node and should be reported.

- You should also report any persistent symptom to the supervising physician, especially bone pain, cough, shortness of breath, persistent abdominal pain.

The reason for this intensive attention to detail is not to turn you into someone preoccupied with illness. In fact, all the procedures of good follow-up care after breast surgery can be taken care of in a relatively short time. The point is simple: the investment can be really important to your well-being.

CHAPTER

13

RECURRENCE

L ife is often not fair, and the recurrence of a cancer you thought had been safely beaten back and destroyed is particularly hard to take. Who could keep from worrying about survival and dreading the prospect of a new round of treatment?

These emotions are completely understandable and there is no easy way to explain why any particular person becomes ill again. The risks of recurrence of breast cancer have gone way down in recent years, and as we will see in the chapter on new research, there is reason to hope that those risks can be even further reduced. Unfortunately, however, as of this moment, even with the best treatment and the most meticulous follow-up care, cancer may recur.

What to do now? Haven't you already used all available resources?

By no means. Fortunately, of all carcinomas, breast cancer is one of the most sensitive to treatment. There is a large array of treatments that can be called upon to bring the illness under control and to permit women to live normal lives, often for many years, even after recurrence.

What is required—from both the patient and the physician—is a determined effort, a forceful attack. And that brings us to the crucial first step in treating a recurrence of breast cancer:

FINDING THE RIGHT DOCTOR

You have read that many times before in this book. In Chapter Two and elsewhere, we've discussed the crucial importance of the right physician at every step along the way. But it is at this juncture, when there has been a recurrence, that the task of choosing someone to manage your case is especially subtle and especially important.

Why is this choice an issue yet again? Why shouldn't you just continue with the physician who has been handling your case up to now, the one who has been acting—with your agreement—as the leader or coordinator of the team of doctors you've been seeing?

Despite the recurrence, there is a good chance that going back to one of the doctors who originally treated you is an excellent thing to do. Nevertheless, even if all you want is the reassurance of a fresh evaluation, you should certainly get more than one opinion. It makes sense to reevaluate the work of the people who were responsible for your care and to consider alternatives. You may eventually decide to find a new "leader" to work with, or you may decide to remain with one or more of the doctors on the original team. But because a recurrence poses special risks, you will need a doctor who is thoroughly familiar with what has been called the natural history of cancer.

He should have treated many patients with recurring breast cancer so that he understands the hazards that may lie ahead and the steps that must be taken to avoid them.

His approach should be vigorous. That does not mean he should rush into therapies that are unnecessarily harsh or risky. It does involve a quality we referred to in Chapter Two: particularly at this stage of the illness, you want someone who will approach the disease as an impassioned advocate, determined to secure the best possible outcome for you.

The art of diagnosis is especially important in dealing with a recurrence. Look for a doctor who is meticulous and who will have the time and the patience both to analyze what is wrong with you and to seek out the latest information on the treatment that is most appropriate for your condition.

New techniques are constantly being developed. The physician you pick should present you with a state-of-the-art treatment plan, tailored specifically to your needs.

In order to do this, he should be up-to-the-minute on the latest research so that he can incorporate proven new approaches into your treatment. But he should use such treatment not because it is "the latest thing" but because there is strong reason to believe that it will benefit you.

Though a recurrence should be fought aggressively, the doctor must bear in mind that you are not only a patient, but also a person with a life to live, with your own interests and responsibilities. The treatment plan must take that into account. The aim should be to provide the most effective care possible; to try to limit side effects; and to give treatment that is consistent with your expressed wishes so that you can continue as much as possible to lead the kind of life you prefer.

HOW DO YOU FIND SUCH A PERSON?

1. Concentrate first on who would be the primary doctor, the one who coordinates the team. This should be someone whose opinion you trust, to whom you can talk freely, and who is good at what he does.

2. Review the sections in Chapter Two on finding and choosing a doctor.

3. Consult the sections that follow on what background material the physician should ask for and what your first meeting with him should be like. If the new physician

does not seem to cover thoroughly all the points we mention, or if his judgments don't strike you as thoughtful and confident, you should probably look elsewhere.

WHAT TO TAKE WITH YOU TO THE CONSULTANT'S OFFICE

Whether you are going for another opinion or seeking a new manager of your case, you will have to bring with you to the consultation as much information as possible, so the physician can fully understand your previous illness and how it was treated.

There is no doctor I know who doesn't get a twinge in whatever part of his anatomy his pride resides when a patient announces that she wants to consult someone else. But a competent and compassionate physician will recognize that when you are confronted with a serious medical problem, you should make as sure as possible that you are doing the right thing. The consultation may well result in your staying with your own doctor, reassured that the proposed plan of treatment makes sense. Perhaps the original medical team and the consultant may confer on your condition. Maybe you will decide to change physicians. What you should always remember is that it's your well-being that is at stake and your choice about how best to protect it.

Here are the things the consulting physician should ask for and that you should try to take with you to your first appointment:

1. A letter from your primary physician summarizing what has happened in your case up until the present. (Allow time for the letter to be prepared.)

2. A copy of the original surgery report, called an operative report. This detailed report of exactly what was done during the procedure is prepared by the surgeon and is part of the hospital record. Copies are kept in the surgeon's office.

3. Similar reports of any later operations or biopsies. These are available in the surgeon's office.

4. For each surgery and biopsy, there should be an accompanying pathology report. Many doctors will also ask you to bring them the actual slides of the tissue sections that were examined by the pathologist. The surgeon will have the pathology report, and his nurse can tell you how to get the slides if you need them.

5. If you had radiation therapy, ask the radiologist for a radiation therapy report that summarizes the doses and the fields to which radiation was administered.

6. Sometimes the consulting physician will want reports on tests and treatments that were done in the hospital. Usually, the easiest way to get these is by using a request-for-records form. The consulting physician's office should send this form, signed by you, to the hospital's medical records department. The reports will then be sent to the consultant's office. You can also obtain such reports yourself at most hospitals, but the procedure is more complicated. In both cases, a fee may be charged.

7. The films of X rays and scans may be at your radiologist's office or at the hospital. To get these from the hospital, the consulting physician's office must usually fill out another request-for-records form. Sign the form and have it marked with a statement that says, "Give material to patient or family member, please." Then you or someone you choose can pick up the material either from the file room of the hospital's X-ray department or from another file room to which X-ray department personnel can direct you. There is sometimes a charge for this service.

A COMPANION

It is a good idea to take someone with you when you discuss your recurrence with the doctors you consult. Refer to Chapter Six for advice on choosing a personal advocate.

Ask the help of that person and others who are close to you in getting all the material you need from previous doctors and the hospital. Try to spare yourself having to do these chores on your own.

With the assistance of your companion and any others who may be of help to you, prepare a list of questions before your appointment. Give a copy of the list to the companion who accompanies you to the doctor's office and ask her to take the responsibility for making sure all your concerns are covered.

Ask your companion to take notes during your office visits of what the doctor says and of any instructions he gives you.

THE FIRST VISIT TO THE CONSULTANT

1. The physician should carefully explore with you the discovery of the recurrence:

   • Did you find a new symptom or sign of illness yourself?

   • What was the symptom or sign? A new lump? Pain anywhere in the body? An inflammation of the skin?

   • Did the recurrence show up on one of your follow-up tests? Which one?

   • Since the discovery, has a biopsy been performed? What were the pathologist's findings?

   • Have other tests been performed? What were their results?

2. The physician should now take a complete medical history. (See Chapter Fourteen.)

3. A thorough physical examination should be performed, as described in Chapter Two.

4. Though the records you have brought with you may provide enough information for the consultant to recommend a treatment plan, there is the possibility that he may feel it necessary to order new tests in order to confirm the diagnosis of recurrence and also to measure its extent. Good

decisions will rely on answers to such questions as: Is the recurrence only in one area of the body? More than one?

5. With such information, the doctor will confirm the diagnosis, assess the extent of the disease, and establish a baseline, a summary of the current status of the illness that can be used to evaluate how you respond to later treatment.

6. After the diagnosis, you and the consultant should be able to discuss tentative treatment options. The actual treatment plan may have to be taken up at a later visit, after all the information has been analyzed, and when you have decided who will supervise your care.

7. At this time, the consultant will usually report his findings and treatment suggestions to your primary physician. It is at this point that you may have to decide whether to continue with your current primary physician or to choose someone else to manage your treatment.

WHERE IS THE RECURRENCE?

When cancer cells leave their site of origin, that is, when they metastasize, they must find a hospitable environment. In order to survive, cancer cells require a type of tissue to which they can adhere and the formation of blood vessels that will bring them nutrition.

Because of their particular properties, breast cancer cells are most likely to establish themselves and produce a tumor recurrence in bone. Though any part of the skeleton may be affected, some bones are more likely to be involved than others. The bones of the spine, ribs, pelvis, and upper parts of the arms and legs are frequent sites; the bones of the arm below the elbow or of the leg below the knee are seldom affected.

Breast cancer may also spread into the skin and the lymph nodes. Among other organ systems, the lungs and liver are the most likely sites of recurrence.

In order to plan the treatment, we have to find out whether

the recurrence is local or distant. A local recurrence is limited to the area of the previous surgery. Has the cancer come back in a breast previously treated with lumpectomy and radiation? In the chest wall at the site of a previous mastectomy?

A recurrence is considered distant if it is any place in the body other than the breast or the chest wall of the previously treated area. It is considered distant even if it is relatively close to the original site, above the collarbone, for example.

PROGNOSIS

People with recurrences are sometimes told that though long-term control of the cancer is possible, there are no cures of recurrent breast cancer. *There are an increasing number of exceptions to this so-called rule.*

The goal in each case should be to strive to make the particular patient who is being treated an exception to the rule. If it turns out that we cannot achieve that goal, then, after fighting the cancer with all our resources, we must see to it that every patient survives as long as possible.

I have seen many women go on, after a recurrence, to live a fulfilling life:

The wife of a childhood friend came to me many years ago with a local recurrence in the chest wall after mastectomy. At that time, her risk for a series of increasingly serious recurrences was extremely high. We had two choices: to use standard treatment and then wait for the inevitable; or to use the then relatively new combination chemotherapy in an all-out effort to achieve a cure. After discussion with the patient, the cancer was removed and the chest wall was treated with radiation. (We would now also prescribe tamoxifen, but since we didn't have the drug then, we removed the woman's ovaries.) I then began to treat her with chemotherapy, not knowing how long such treatment should continue. When the first year was over, I agonized over the risks of going on and of adding another group of drugs, and I finally decided to go ahead for another two years. It's fifteen years later now and my friend is still well.

Another patient had extensive recurrences in her chest wall. Surgery and radiation had been tried in the two years before she came to see me, and they had failed. The recurrences kept appearing and she now had pain, suggesting a bone cancer. The family was told that the patient had less than a year to live.

CMFVP (see page 175) was still an experimental treatment at the time, but we started using it and, to our joy, complete remission was achieved within ten months. To maintain the remission, I continued treating this woman for three years before we stopped. She lived a full life, saw her children marry, and enjoyed her grandchildren, before, still free of cancer, she died of another cause fourteen years later.

There are many more stories like these, some of them bittersweet but still important. For example, a young woman called me recently to tell me that her mother, whom I had treated many years before for breast cancer, had recently died of a cancer in the lung. The daughter had only been three years old when her mother came to the office with an inoperable, extensive recurrence of cancer at the mastectomy site. Radiation therapy and three years of chemotherapy kept her cancer-free for sixteen years. Then she apparently developed a tumor in the lung, was treated conservatively, and died two years later. I felt a great sadness at this news, but her daughter had another view: she was actually calling to thank me for "giving her a mother" during her childhood.

The point of these histories? Sometimes we don't understand why a patient with a serious diagnosis seems to defy the odds and go on living a good life. We don't always know why the disease may be in remission, that is, inactive for many years. Prognosis, as we learned in Chapter Nine, is a prediction, one that is dependent on statistics and not necessarily applicable to any particular individual. And most important in considering recurrence—with vigorous, determined therapy, the odds can be made to tilt in your favor.

TREATMENT

Local Recurrences

If the original breast cancer was treated with lumpectomy and it has reappeared only in the treated breast, this does not mean that the disease has spread. It indicates either a recurrence in that spot or a new cancer in another part of the breast.

Surgery is the primary treatment. In most instances, the breast now has to be removed in what you may hear referred to as a salvage mastectomy. Reconstruction is possible but, if radiation was used after the surgery, you will need one of the flap procedures described in Chapter Eleven, rather than an implant.

Chemotherapy and/or hormone therapy is the next step. The regimen to be used will depend on the nature of the test findings and on whether or not you received adjuvant treatment the first time your breast cancer was treated.

If the recurrence is on the chest wall, at the site of the mastectomy, it indicates regrowth of the original cancer and is associated with a higher risk of spread to other parts of the body. Rarely, a new breast cancer may grow in a remnant of breast tissue retained under the mastectomy flaps. This has a lesser risk of spread.

Surgery is the first step, with the removal of the cancer. A margin of healthy tissue must also be removed. Depending on the size of the tumor and its location, this may involve removing underlying muscle and possibly bone; or it may only require a fairly limited excision.

To make sure that any microscopic disease in the area is destroyed, radiation is administered to the entire region of the mastectomy.

A course of hormone therapy or chemotherapy follows, though it has not been established whether this treatment should continue for limited or prolonged periods of time. My own practice is to treat women with a recurrence in the chest wall as though they have had a recurrence in a distant part of the body. There have been enough women in my own practice who have fared well with this program that I consider this an instance where, at times, recurrent cancer may be cured.

Distant Recurrences

I want to talk now about the word *palliate,* which the *Random House Dictionary* defines as "to relieve or lessen without curing." Palliation is the goal of many oncologists who treat recurrent breast cancer. They want to help their patients, of course, but because they believe that a recurrence is the signal that a patient will not survive, their goal is to palliate, to treat the disease as best they can without causing too many unpleasant side effects or discomfort.

Since there are now so many options for the treatment of breast cancer through hormone therapy and chemotherapy, almost all patients can expect palliation of their disease. But, difficult as it may be, many of us do not automatically accept palliation as a goal. We look at each case individually and try to devise a strategy that achieves more than that. Sometimes, such a strategy may involve using a program likely to produce significant side effects. Those must be measured against the risks of the disease and the potential benefits of the treatment.

Given this philosophy, which I share, how do we treat recurrences at distant sites? With the weapons now at our disposal: surgery, radiation, hormone therapy, and chemotherapy.

1. For disease that has spread, surgery is used to remove an isolated tumor or other cancerous tissue that gets in the way of normal function.

2. In cases where there is an isolated metastasis—a site in the lung or brain, for example—we can at times provide a cure by removing it.

3. Radiation can reach otherwise-hard-to-get-at locations, and it is particularly useful in relieving pain in bones where cancer has metastasized. It can destroy tumors in parts of the body that you would not want to interfere with surgically, and it also works fairly quickly.

4. Hormone therapy can be used for women who have hormone-positive receptors (see pages 86–87). It seems to work particularly well for women who have been free of cancer for a relatively long time since breast surgery, who have bone and soft tissue involvement rather than disease

of the liver or lung, who reacted well to previous hormone therapy.

5. For some patients, very-high-dose chemotherapy followed by bone-marrow and/or stem-cell transplant (see pages 175–176) offers a chance for cure.

(See Chapter Ten for descriptions of many of the drugs that are referred to below, including their side effects. Only drugs new to this chapter are described here.)

Women with recurrent tumors that are both estrogen- and progesterone-receptor positive respond to hormone treatment in almost seventy-five percent of cases. When only one type of hormone receptor is present, the response falls to forty percent, and to ten percent when both receptor levels are negative.

The first hormone-related drug used is almost always tamoxifen. Used alone, it can be very effective even in advanced breast cancer, but unfortunately, it stops working, on average, in a little over a year. The physician can, however, usually switch to another drug and get a satisfactory response.

The drug often used next is aminoglutethemide (Cytadren), which acts to reduce the estrogen-like products of the adrenal gland. Because this drug also lowers the body's production of cortisone, an essential hormone, a cortisone supplement is usually given with it. The major side effect, sleepiness, can be alleviated if you start with a low dose. If you take the medication with food, you can avoid gastric irritation; and the oral form of cortisone forestalls a possible rash that may appear if the aminoglutethemide is given alone. Drugs similar to aminoglutethemide that are more specific for suppressing estrogen production (aromatase inhibitors) are beginning to appear. Anastrozole (Arimidex) is the first of this group to be approved by the FDA.

When the effectiveness of this drug fails, an agent that resembles a male hormone, usually Halotestin, may sometimes be used. This drug is said to be particularly effective for treating bone metastases.

Megestrol (Megace), a progesterone-like substance, is also commonly used in hormone therapy. It increases appetite and therefore causes weight gain.

Leuprolide (Lupron), a newly available drug, mimics a natural hormone that decreases pituitary function and thus reduces estrogen levels. It is well-tolerated by most patients, though a long list of side effects has been reported.

Hormone treatment plays an important role in the treatment of recurrent breast cancer. Unfortunately, each drug has to be given in sequence because, in time, it will stop being effective. It is for this reason that we prefer to combine hormone treatment with chemotherapy. In fact, even for patients who are hormone-receptor positive and who respond to hormone therapy, there is some evidence that when the two therapies are combined, better results may be obtained.

Chemotherapy

If the original tumor or the recurring tumor has no hormone receptors, chemotherapy is used from the beginning of the treatment, always in combinations of drugs. If the patient's tumor is receptor-positive, many oncologists, myself included, combine chemotherapy with hormone therapy.

The first chemotherapy program used for a recurrence, in what is called first-line therapy, uses drug combinations that contain either methotrexate or Adriamycin. (Refer to Chapter Ten for a full discussion of the drugs and drug combinations used in chemotherapy.)

Typical alternatives are CMF, CMFVP, CAF, or FAC. Nearly all these combinations produce responses in fifty to sixty percent of patients. CMF works for about eight months on average, the other combinations for about one year each, though both much longer and shorter periods of effectiveness also occur.

If an Adriamycin-based program was used for the first line, the next regimen, the second-line therapy, will use a methotrexate-based program, and vice versa. If one of these was used for adjuvant treatment before the recurrence, the other will now be used. The term *third-line* is used to describe the regimens that are used next.

Drug combinations are always in development and research is likely to yield new programs at any time. Major advances have been made in recent years with the introduction of new second- and third-line treatments. They involve some of the drugs we've already discussed as well as a few others:

233

- **Leucovorin** was at one time used primarily to limit the side effects of methotrexate. It is now also used to make 5-fluorouracil more effective.

- **Mitomycin-C** (Mutamycin) is a natural product that interferes with DNA synthesis. It is most often used as a third-line treatment in combination with vinblastine.

- **Mitoxantrone** (Novantrone) works by a process that eventually inactivates DNA. It resembles Adriamycin in both therapeutic efficacy and toxicity.

- **Vinblastine** is related to vincristine, but it may be effective even if vincristine has already been used.

- **Vinorelbine** (Navelbine) is a semisynthetic product of the same plant that is the source of both vincristine and vinblastine. It interferes with the assembly of tubules needed for cell division.

- **Paclitaxel** (Taxol) is another natural product. Although it can now be prepared synthetically, its original source was the bark of the Pacific yew tree. It promotes assembly of the cell tubules needed for cell division, but in an abnormal way, so that affected cells can no longer divide.

- **Docetaxel** (Taxotere), a drug similar to Taxol, is a product of the bark of the European yew tree. It may be effective at times in patients who have not benefited from Taxol.

HOW ARE THESE DRUGS USED?

Here is a summary of the principles that guide the use of chemotherapy for recurrent disease.

- When several treatment alternatives are available, the one selected should be the one that is likely to produce the greatest degree of tumor destruction.

- Since treatment benefits tend to diminish after a period of time, if two treatments produce equal levels of tumor destruction, the preferred treatment is the one that, on the average, is able to maintain tumor control longer.

- For maximum benefit, whenever possible chemotherapy should be integrated with other forms of treatment, such as surgery and radiation, to reduce each patient's tumor burden to a minimum.

- Combinations of drugs are generally more effective than single drugs in treating breast cancer.
- Strategies to minimize and overcome side effects should be part of every treatment plan.

COMMONLY USED TREATMENTS

The most commonly used first- and second-line combinations, CMF, CMFVP, CAF, and FAC, have been discussed in Chapter 10 (see pages 174, 175). The following are additional treatment programs:

- **Leucovorin, 5-fluorouracil** is a third-line treatment that now seems the most effective. The drugs are given in sequence, with leucovorin always first. Leucovorin is referred to as a 5-fluorouracil modulator because it significantly increases the effectiveness of a drug that by itself has only a modest effect on breast cancer.
- **Methotrexate, 5-fluorouracil, and leucovorin** is another program that is useful in high doses. The high-dose methotrexate also acts as a modulator to enhance the effects of the 5-fluorouracil, but leucovorin must be taken eighteen to twenty hours later, to stop the methotrexate action and limit its side effects. This program often works even after leucovorin, 5-fluorouracil has failed.
- **5-fluorouracil** by continuous infusion requires placement of an Infus-a-Port or similar device (see page 168) to permit ready access to the venous circulation. 5-fluorouracil is then given intravenously through the Infus-a-Port, using a small pump that is worn in a pouch at belt level. Depending on the doses used, the drug can be given uninterruptedly for twenty-four hours a day for several days, for three weeks, or for months.
- **Adriamycin, Taxol** as a combination may be effective in situations where either drug alone gives limited benefit.
- **VATH** is used for patients who have failed methotrexate-containing combinations. It is unique in combining chemotherapy with the hormone Halotestin.

- **Mitoxantrone, Thiotepa, with or without methotrexate,** is a drug combination that is useful for third-line therapy if only limited amounts of Adriamycin have previously been used.

- **Mitomycin-C, vinblastine** was at one time considered to be the standard third-line treatment. Though it is still in use, it is not likely to be effective in patients who have previously received large amounts of vincristine or Adriamycin.

- **Taxol** is effective even for advanced disease. However, its benefits are not always long-lasting. In addition to combining Taxol with other drugs, alternate schedules of administration are being tried to increase its efficacy. Studies are under way of Taxol given over a period of 96 hours, or in smaller weekly doses.

- **Taxotere and Navelbine** are newer drugs that have shown promising antitumor effects in early clinical studies. While they may ultimately prove to be important new agents for the treatment of breast cancer, their value remains to be determined by more comprehensive clinical trials.

Using the principles outlined above for choosing which of these programs to use at a given time to treat a patient with recurrent disease, the skilled medical oncologist bases his treatment both on published studies of relative efficacy and on his own experience. It is reassuring that breast cancer does respond to a wide range of treatments.

SIDE EFFECTS

Side effects common to many forms of chemotherapy have been discussed in Chapter 10 (see pages 176–183). Here are details of specific side effects of the drugs and combinations we have mentioned.

- **Leucovorin** is a derivative of a B vitamin, folic acid. Leucovorin may produce an allergic reaction, but otherwise has no major side effects.

- **Mitomycin-C** can injure the kidney and lung. It causes

blood-count changes, which may persist. If it is accidentally released under the skin, it may cause major damage.

- **Vinblastine** produces more blood-count suppression and causes less nerve damage than vincristine.

- **Vinorelbine** causes marked declines in white-blood-cell counts, which may require Neupogen (see page 179) to correct. Nerve damage, similar to that produced by vincristine, and nausea, are other side effects.

- **Taxol,** in addition to changes in blood count, may produce a severe allergic reaction at the time it is given. All patients must receive treatment with a combination of drugs for twelve hours before Taxol is administered, in order to prevent this response. Nerve damage, nausea, diarrhea, and/or arthritic pain may occur.

- **Taxotere** is similar to Taxol, but causes fluid retention in addition.

- **Mitoxantrone** causes nausea, heart damage, and decreases in blood counts.

- **Thiotepa** causes fatigue, nausea, burning at times on urination, and dizziness.

- **Leucovorin, 5-fluorouracil** may cause burning in the mouth, hyperacidity, and diarrhea. This combination generally has fewer side effects than 5-fluorouracil alone, as long as dosage is carefully controlled.

- **Methotrexate, 5-fluorouracil, and leucovorin** have side effects similar to leucovorin, 5-fluorouracil, but the combination tends to produce greater fatigue.

- **Mitoxantrone, Thiotepa, with or without methotrexate,** causes fatigue, a fall in blood counts, burning mouth, and possible heart damage.

- **Mitomycin, vincristine** causes a fall in blood counts, which may persist. Long-term administration can injure the kidneys.

AUTOLOGOUS BONE-MARROW AND/OR STEM-CELL TRANSPLANT

This new method to support high-dose chemotherapy as a means of achieving cure is now sometimes being used for women with distant metastases. While it is associated with potentially serious side effects, including infections and lung and liver injury, with experience these effects are being significantly reduced. At some centers, transplant therapy is now being performed for suitable patients as an outpatient procedure. Most programs require an initial three months of lower-dose preparatory (or "induction") chemotherapy, followed by one extremely high-dose treatment accompanied by the transplant. This last phase takes three to six weeks to complete. (Refer to page 175 in Chapter Ten for additional discussion of this treatment.) The results of these procedures are still under study, and at this time a bone-marrow transplant regimen is not being given to patients who previously have had multiple treatments, particularly those including Adriamycin.

In the setting of recurrent disease, the greatest promise for this approach is in the treatment of women with a small number of metastatic sites, where chances for long-term benefit are particularly favorable. If bone-marrow transplant is suggested to you, weigh the risks and potential benefits carefully.

FOLLOW-UP DURING THERAPY

You should be carefully examined and tested during your treatment for complications and side effects and to keep track of your general physical condition. (Review in Chapter Ten the steps that should be followed in a visit to the oncologist's office.) We also want to know as precisely as possible whether the treatment is working, whether it is beginning to fail, and when we feel safe in stopping. Careful monitoring allows us to step in quickly to change therapy should a particular program begin to fail. Blood tests, particularly tumor marker tests (see page 216), can indirectly indicate whether the treatment is affecting the tumor. At intervals, imaging examinations such as X ray, CAT scan, and MRI (see Chapter Four) may be performed for a more direct evaluation of how you are doing.

WHAT HAVE WE LEARNED ABOUT TREATING RECURRENCE WITH CHEMOTHERAPY?

The best results are obtained when we hit hard with the initial treatment after a recurrence, so as to destroy as much of the disease as we can—and, if possible, all of it.

We should use everything we have to attack the cancer; that is, surgery, radiation, and/or hormone therapy and chemotherapy, in sequence or in combination.

If, despite our best efforts, the cancer again recurs, it may be because it has become resistant to the drugs in use. We may be able to prevent such a development by alternating different forms of chemotherapy or by refining the use of such techniques as bone-marrow transplant. As more is being understood about the mechanisms that produce drug resistance, new drugs are being developed to overcome it.

IS THERE AN EFFECTIVE STRATEGY TO USE NOW?

The answer to that question depends on your goals. Is your aim to prolong life? Assure a good life quality with limited drug side effects? Achieve cure?

Any sensible person would answer yes to all three questions. The best approach to treating a recurrence of breast cancer is to devise a strategy that reverses the order of those questions and puts the first and primary emphasis, wherever possible, on trying for cure. We attempt to accomplish that goal with a minimum of disruption of the life of the patient but with the understanding that when we are dealing with an aggressive cancer, we must act aggressively.

Let's now take up these goals one by one:

PROLONGING LIFE

Nearly everyone who has a recurrence of breast cancer can now expect that a strategy of treatment will be used that will arrest the illness for a significant period of time. The initial treatment after recurrence is more effective than treatments of the past, and if that treatment fails, there are several alternatives that can be used to restore control of the illness.

239

ASSURING THE QUALITY OF LIFE

The first thing to be said is that the use of chemotherapy is not inconsistent with preserving the quality of a patient's life. As we have seen, some oncologists, whose goal is palliation, do not give chemotherapy to patients with recurrent cancer so as to spare them what they consider "unnecessary suffering." Instead they may use hormone therapy alone as the first treatment after a recurrence, and turn to chemotherapy only after the hormones no longer work. While this may be appropriate in selected cases, my concern is that this approach gives chemotherapy less chance to be effective, because it is not being brought into play until the cancer has further progressed.

Chemotherapy, properly administered, need not cause patients anguish and suffering. The best quality of life, after all, comes from the lasting, complete remission that the early and creative use of chemotherapy may achieve.

CURE

Some patients with recurring breast cancer, particularly those with local recurrences, were cured in the past, but they were the exceptions. In most instances, the disease eventually came back, despite the use of the best treatment then available.

But better strategies are now available. We do not have to accept the history of breast cancer recurrence as its future. The oncologist can examine the treatments now available and devise a specific program that will give each patient the best possible chance.

Does this mean that everyone with recurrent breast cancer will be cured? No. But, in my opinion, a creative, intensive approach certainly increases the length of remission and at the present time actually may cure some women. Over time, with more research, we hope to cure all of them.

CHAPTER

14

PREVENTION

❧

A s we begin to talk about the prevention of breast cancer, we have to say that we don't know much about it. What we do know, however, is that there is no credible evidence to support the idea that women have done something to themselves to cause them to become ill. Your psychological attitude did not give you cancer. It is bad enough to develop cancer without having someone tell you that you have only yourself to blame. It's a burden no one deserves, and the blame really lies on the so-called experts who write books about "cancer personalities," or give simplistic advice about how you can cure yourself with good cheer.

As you will see in Chapter Fifteen on new research, a lot is now going on that may tell us, within the next few years, what causes breast cancer. That is the information we need before we can give definitive advice on how to prevent the disease.

If we knew more, for example, about why being born with a mutant gene places women at risk for developing breast cancer, we could work to find a strategy to correct the problem, perhaps through genetic engineering.

If we knew that the mutant gene triggers breast cancer only under certain environmental or nutritional or other circumstances, we could work to protect women from those triggers.

If we knew why, when breast cancer spreads, it is often to the bone, the liver, and the lungs, and very seldom to the spleen, the kidney, or the skeletal muscle, perhaps then we would be able to develop effective preventive measures.

In the meantime, we have to look at the data that are now available about the incidence of breast cancer and various correlations with risk factors, and try to draw from them whatever lessons we can about prevention.

IS THE INCIDENCE OF BREAST CANCER INCREASING?

There is statistical evidence that it is, and there is certainly a lot of anecdotal evidence. A woman said to me the other day, "I had breast cancer, my sister has it, and three or four people we grew up with are sick. We're all in our fifties, but this week I sent a friend who's thirty-six and about to get married to see you. I have another friend in her forties who has it, and someone in my office who's only twenty-five, and my neighbor's eighty-year-old grandmother. They come from all different backgrounds and they're young and old, Asian and black and white. What is this, an epidemic?"

It's probably not, at this moment, an epidemic by scientific definition, but there is no doubt that breast cancer is on the rise and that the rise is surprisingly high among young women. There are now more than 184,000 new cases of breast cancer every year, more new cases than of any other cancer. There are thirty percent more cases now than there were in the 1970s. One in nine women is expected to develop breast cancer in her lifetime. In 1975, it was one in fifteen. The annual increase is large enough so that it can't be explained away by factors like early detection, or more openness about reporting the disease, or greater publicity. There is simply more breast cancer than ever before.

WHAT IS THE CAUSE OF THE INCREASE?

There are probably several risk factors that make individuals more vulnerable to developing breast cancer. What are they?

It's important to note here that we're not asking, "What can I do to avoid breast cancer?" in every instance. As you will see, several of the risk factors are beyond our control. Furthermore, studies have shown that fifty-five to seventy-five percent of women with breast cancer have no known risk factors. What we are exploring now is whether certain circumstances can be shown to be related to the disease.

Heredity

Eighty-five percent of women who develop breast cancer have no family history whatsoever. Of the remaining fifteen percent, about a third do seem to have a genetic connection, particularly when first-degree maternal relatives have had breast cancer, or they are age forty or younger.

If an aunt or cousin or grandmother had breast cancer, the chance of developing the disease is one and a half times the average. If a mother and sister have had it, the risk is five to six times greater. If they had it in both breasts, the risk increases to five to ten times the average. In such families, breast cancer will tend to occur at an earlier age in succeeding generations, often before menopause.

Does that mean that if there is breast cancer in your family you are certain to get it? No. As with the other risk factors and statistical odds we've been discussing throughout the book, this family history says nothing about any particular individual. Not every woman in such a family is fated for breast cancer. In fact, in studies of identical twins, where you would expect that if one twin gets an illness, the other will invariably get it, too, the second twin does not necessarily get breast cancer.

In the next chapter we will discuss what we are learning about genes that may increase susceptibility to breast cancer.

243

Race

We begin with some numbers that are not, strictly speaking, concerned with the risk of developing breast cancer. They do, however, have a lot to do with the risk of not surviving the disease. While the incidence of breast cancer is a little lower for black women than for white, once they get the disease, African-American women do not do nearly as well. In fact, their survival rate dropped by fourteen percent in the 1980s; the survival rate actually increased for white women in the same period.

Why? It probably has a lot to do with poverty. One-third of all Americans are, by common definition, poor. One-third of the poor are black. Many African-Americans—as well as other economically disadvantaged women—cannot afford mammography, professional physical examination, and other health care, and therefore come for treatment when the disease has advanced beyond the early stages. About seventy percent of black women have never had a mammogram. In addition, many of our public health facilities have a woeful record in treating poor women. In New York City it was reported recently that a third of those who are surgically treated for breast cancer in public hospitals received no further treatment.

So, the risk of developing breast cancer is not worse for black women than for others. It is the risk of their surviving the illness that American society must begin to address.

In the past, Asian women had a lower breast cancer rate than Caucasians. Prior to World War II, for example, the disease was very uncommon in Japan. Then it was noticed that the rate began to rise in Japanese women who had emigrated to Hawaii. And when the daughters of these women were born and raised in Hawaii, their incidence of breast cancer was the same as the native-born Caucasian population. (And white Hawaiian women have among the highest breast cancer rates in the world!)

Is there something about the air or water in Hawaii that causes breast cancer? Who knows? What we do know is that first-generation Japanese women living in San Francisco had a three-fold rise in breast cancer over the women who stayed in Japan. And the sad development of recent years is that since 1975, the breast cancer rate has risen enormously in Japan as well. We can only speculate on the reasons for this phenomenon, but here are some of the possibilities:

244

- The Japanese diet has been "Westernized" to include a lot more fat than it had before, particularly animal fat.
- Japanese women have begun to menstruate earlier and to enter menopause later than those before World War II.
- Japanese women now marry later and have their first child later than was customary in the past.
- The environment has changed a great deal in Japan just as it has in the rest of the world. Greatly increased industrialization has brought with it sharply increased air pollution and other environmental hazards.

Diet

The most plausible culprit in the Japanese breast cancer mystery would seem to be the radical change in diet. The possibility that a high-calorie diet, and particularly a high consumption of fat, is connected to breast cancer has been supported by the kinds of studies we have been discussing, epidemiologic studies that compare large populations of people. It has been supported as well by laboratory experiments with animals.

A "special communication" from the *Journal of the American Medical Association* in 1989 said, "Data from animal experiments and human correlation studies strongly support the dietary fat—breast cancer hypothesis. . . . Animals fed a high-fat, high-calorie diet have a substantially higher incidence of mammary tumors than animals fed a low-fat, calorie-restricted diet."

Additionally, we know that, particularly in postmenopausal women, fat cells play a role in the production of estrogen. As we will see, there is reason to believe that a long period of estrogen stimulation is linked to breast cancer. Postmenopausal women who are overweight produce more estrogen and would therefore benefit from a lower-calorie diet.

Though not all population studies have supported this hypothesis about diet, there is very little to be lost from taking your cue from these data and lowering fat and calorie intake. By one estimate, a woman on a typical American diet could reduce her risk of getting breast cancer by

- lowering fat intake to less than twenty percent of the calories she consumes

245

- lowering saturated-fat intake to less than ten percent
- lowering intake of animal proteins to less than six percent

There are many people around the country who go further than this and advocate much more radical diet changes. A diet composed primarily of complex carbohydrates is said both to prevent cancer and to play a role in its cure. The same kinds of claims are made for macrobiotic diets.

All that can be said at this point is that there is no convincing evidence that such drastic regimens do what their proponents claim. A prudent diet rich in complex carbohydrates and fiber and low in fats is undoubtedly better for you than a diet rich in simple sugars and fats. But it does not seem sensible to eliminate from your diet other foods that may be useful to your body. Not enough is known about the effects of severely restricted diets for us to be able to say that they don't do more harm than good.

Vitamins and Minerals

As with the claims for radically limited diets, there is no evidence that megadoses of vitamins and minerals decrease the risk of breast cancer. In fact, it seems to be our best-nourished women who are at greatest risk for breast cancer. While it is true that such women probably eat more fat than they should, their diets are also rich in vitamins and minerals.

Foods that are replete with vitamins and minerals are essential to your well-being. It may also be good for you to take moderate amounts of supplemental vitamins. Some of these supplements—calcium in postmenopausal women, for example—do seem to have beneficial effects. But taking too much of a particular vitamin or mineral supplement can be dangerous, and there are documented cases of severe side effects. If you have been discovered through good, credible tests to have a deficiency, you should almost certainly use vitamin or mineral supplements, but self-medication can be harmful. Not all anemias, for example, are caused by iron deficiencies. In fact, the storage of excess iron in the body can lead to all sorts of unpleasant and even dangerous side effects.

Furthermore, some of the media "stars" among these supplements seem to perform poorly. The cancer protection afforded by selenium, for example, had been widely touted in the press, but a very convincing study refutes these claims. And, on the other side of the coin, there have been a few reported fatalities from taking contaminated selenium.

Alcohol

There is continuing investigation of the link between drinking and breast cancer. A recent study seemed to show some correlation with moderate drinking, but that study has been criticized. At the moment, nothing very definite can be said that translates into breast cancer prevention.

Caffeine

There is no indication, at the present time, that there is any link between caffeine and breast cancer. Coffee, tea, colas, and chocolate all contain caffeine, and though there was said to be some correlation between consuming these substances and developing breast cysts, the connection has not been proved. Some women whose breasts tend to become tender and lumpy during their menstrual periods report that limiting their intake of caffeine seems to help, but many more notice no link.

You don't need caffeine to be healthy, so if it makes you feel better to cut it out, there's no reason not to. But there is no evidence that it poses a cancer risk.

Smoking

Lung cancer has become the number-one cancer-killer of women in the United States, exceeding breast cancer. That is a maddening tragedy because lung cancer, with its poor cure rate, is a disease we do know how to prevent. If women would stop smoking, most of them would not get lung cancer. Smoking does not, however, cause breast cancer. It does limit the ways in which we can treat the disease (see Chapter Eleven), since certain surgical reconstruction procedures cannot be used for women who smoke.

Radiation Exposure

Exposure to low or modest levels of radiation may cause breast cancer. (See pages 147–148 for a fuller discussion.)

Young adult women who were exposed to radiation at Hiroshima were subsequently followed and were found to develop an increased number of breast tumors.

Women who were treated with upper-body radiation in the past have been found to have an increased risk of breast cancer.

Although you are exposed to relatively little radiation in any single diagnostic X ray, repeated X rays over a long period of time may increase your cancer risk, particularly at the site of radiation.

As we saw in previous chapters, modern mammography requires very little radiation. Make sure that the mammography facility you go to has been certified by the Food and Drug Administration. (See pages 58–60.)

Other Environmental Causes

We simply don't have any definite cause-and-effect conclusions to offer on this question. We do know that there seem to be geographic "hot spots" for breast cancer as there are for several other cancers; that is, there are certain areas of the United States where, for reasons we often don't completely understand, there is a higher incidence of an illness than would ordinarily be expected.

We have read, for example, of the high rate of blood cancers in parts of New Jersey and of breast cancer on Long Island, and one can hypothesize about the causes. The only thing, however, that can definitely be said about breast cancer and environmental hazards is that a lot more study should be funded and carried out as soon as possible.

Hormones

There seem to be some quite striking connections between breast cancer and hormones and, by extension, between breast cancer and the course of your reproductive life. This is one of a group of risk factors we alluded to at the beginning of this chapter—the ones that are frustrating because there's not much you can do about them.

Perhaps, when more research is done, we will understand better, for example, the link between breast cancer and estrogen and will be able to apply what we have learned to breast cancer prevention. At the moment, all we can say is that there does seem to be a link. There is a higher breast cancer rate for women who begin menstruating at an early age and who reach menopause at a relatively late age. And women who have an early natural menopause or who are fairly young when they have their ovaries removed also have a lower breast cancer risk.

There are other aspects of a woman's reproductive life that affect breast cancer statistics:

- Never having had a child increases your risk of breast cancer.
- The age at which you had your first child influences your risk. Women whose first child was born before they were eighteen have one-third the risk of developing breast cancer of those whose first child was born after they were thirty-five. Pregnancy before thirty appears to offer some protection against breast cancer.

What seems to be at work here is the body's natural production of estrogen—and, perhaps, progesterone. Women who menstruate for a relatively long portion of their lives have estrogen stimulation regularly during that time and this may be a factor in breast cancer development. About the pregnancy factor, we are less sure. Perhaps it is the high levels of progesterone during pregnancy that offer some protection.

If there is such a connection, what about prescribed hormones, birth control pills, and hormone replacement therapy after menopause?

BIRTH CONTROL PILLS

Birth control pills used to contain large amounts of estrogen, sometimes alone, sometimes together with small amounts of progesterone. In recent years, the two drugs have almost invariably been combined and lower doses have been found to be effective.

Some reports have suggested that long-term use of the Pill may eventually place a woman at greater risk for breast cancer. Other reports have suggested that pills with a high estrogen component pose a problem. However, there have also been studies that show no risk.

This is a personal call. Obviously, you're going to take the Pill—a most effective birth control method—if you feel that the problems or dangers associated with pregnancy outweigh any possible increment in breast cancer risk.

HORMONE REPLACEMENT THERAPY

Estrogen, with or without progesterone, may be used for post-menopausal women

- to alleviate symptoms of menopause like hot flashes and vaginal dryness
- to help prevent osteoporosis, a condition that sometimes afflicts older women, causing their bones to become brittle and to fracture easily

There are also some recent data suggesting that women who were given estrogen replacement therapy over an extended period seemed to suffer fewer heart attacks than women who did not receive the treatment.

Nevertheless, we must look carefully at whether it is sensible for all postmenopausal women to use hormone replacement:

- If you have very troublesome menopausal symptoms, there may be no harm in carefully monitored hormone replacement therapy.
- If, in your particular situation, there is an overwhelming risk of osteoporosis, you should consider the treatment.

You should, however, be cautious. Estrogen does not cause breast cancer, but if cancer is present, estrogen may stimulate its growth. Be sure to have a thorough breast examination before beginning any hormone replacement therapy. And do not take

hormones automatically, simply because you have reached menopause.

Though we don't have all the answers about the use of these
supplements, the following factors should be considered:

- Women with a serious family history of breast cancer
  should try to avoid hormone supplements.
- Women who have breast cysts and find that more cysts
  develop when they start taking estrogen should stop.
- Unless they have had a hysterectomy (surgical removal of
  the uterus), women taking hormone replacement therapy
  are generally advised to use progesterone as well as estrogen because of the possibility of developing uterine cancer.

Why bother with supplemental hormones at all?

- If you know, because of family history or for other reasons,
  that you are at significant risk for osteoporosis, the evidence is quite strong that estrogen replacement will act to
  protect you.
- If you have persisting, troublesome menopausal symptoms, as some women do, you will certainly get relief if you
  use hormone replacement therapy.

Should you take these medications, as a vaginal cream or by
mouth, if you have already had breast cancer? With rare exceptions, the answer has to be "no."

TAMOXIFEN

Women who have taken tamoxifen (see Chapter Ten) as treatment
for breast cancer seem to have a lower incidence of cancer developing in the opposite breast than women who haven't taken this
"antiestrogen" drug.

A Breast Cancer Prevention Trial is now underway to determine whether, in fact, long-term use of tamoxifen may be an
excellent way to prevent breast cancer for high-risk women, such
as those with a strong family history or who have lobular carcinoma *in situ*.

PROPHYLACTIC MASTECTOMIES

This very idea strikes most people as a gruesome suggestion. Have a mastectomy or a bilateral mastectomy even before cancer is found?

To do so is a very serious decision. This approach, however, has been used over the years, particularly for women who have an extremely high risk of developing breast cancer and who are extremely fearful of that possibility. Often, women who elect to have such single or double mastectomies also choose to have breast reconstruction. The procedure may be considered for women

- who have a very serious family history of breast cancer, including a mother or sister who has died of the disease. Genetic tests (see pages 256–257) are becoming available to determine who is at highest risk.

- who have undergone several breast biopsies so that the breast is severely deformed

- whose mammograms show findings that are increasingly difficult to interpret

- whose breast biopsies do not indicate cancer but do show severe cell atypia (see page 43), a strong risk factor

What do I tell my patients? There are a few precautions we can be very definite about. Keep your weight down. Lower fat and caloric intake. Take calcium supplements if you are postmenopausal. Exercise because this is important to weight control. Use self-examination, regularly scheduled mammograms, professional physical examinations, and good follow-up care after you've had cancer.

And I tell people not to smoke. Not because it has much to do with breast cancer, but because there's not much point to breast cancer precautions or any other lifesaving techniques if you're going to die of a smoking connection—lung cancer or heart disease or emphysema.

There is, of course, one recurrent theme in this chapter, as you have no doubt noticed. We really do not know much about prevention, about the specifics of what you should and should not do to keep yourself free of breast cancer. What is urgently needed is research not only on cure, but on the causes and prevention of the disease.

15

NEW
DIRECTIONS

Those of us who are old enough remember when, years ago, the March of Dimes campaign turned the search for a cure for polio into an annual national crusade. The imagination of the entire country was engaged. People went from door to door soliciting contributions, and the scientists who worked in the field and eventually found a vaccine were national heroes. And the effort worked! In a surprisingly short time, the polio epidemics that had been so dreaded came to an end.

Why isn't there a comparable fervor about finding a cure for cancer? In part, perhaps it is because the man who was President of the United States, Franklin D. Roosevelt, was a victim of the disease and a constant, visible symbol of its devastating effects. Also, infantile paralysis, as it was often called, struck down large numbers of children, and that evoked a special sympathy.

But I think that something else is going on as well. Despite the valiant efforts of the American Cancer Society and other organizations, we just don't have the optimism that prevailed when the country marched against polio. Most people don't seem to believe that cancer can be cured. They are wrong. We are making progress in the laboratory in unraveling the puzzle of what unleashes uncontrolled cell growth. We are also making progress in treating the disease. But we could be moving much faster if only we could rally the nation in support of a powerful research effort.

Ralph Waldo Emerson said, "Enthusiasm is one of the most powerful engines of success. When you do a thing, do it with all your might. Put your soul into it . . . and you will accomplish your object. Nothing great was ever achieved without enthusiasm."

In the field of cancer research, there is already a lot to be enthusiastic about in the findings of those who do laboratory research as well as of those who study patients.

MOLECULAR BIOLOGY

This branch of science is concerned with cell function and genetic information, and it is extremely important in cancer research. A most promising area of that research is the burgeoning exploration of the nature of genes. Almost every week we learn more about normal genes as well as those implicated in cancer. This research is moving so fast that there is a good chance that its results may be translated very soon into techniques of cancer prevention and treatment.

In order to understand what is going on, it may be helpful to review the nature of cells, chromosomes, and genes, if only enough to be able to interpret the many reports of new discoveries in this field and their application to cancer.

Cells and Computers

We want to concentrate here not on the use of computers in research, but on the computer as a good model for understanding how the human cell works.

For a computer to function, it must rely on stored instructions that can be called upon for solutions to specific problems. These instructions are written in a language the computer can "read." The human cell also works from stored instructions, but they are written in another sort of language—the genetic code. Computer instructions are stored in programs, each with a specific task. The equivalent units in the cells, complex and efficient programs, are called genes.

The computer stores its information on a disk. The coded information of the human cell is stored in meticulously organized structures called chromosomes. Despite its microscopic size, each human cell contains more stored instructions than the largest supercomputer now in use.

To use a computer, you first have to instruct it to call upon a specific program. In order to do that, you type onto the screen, for example, "WordPerfect" or "Lotus." To receive program instructions, the cells have receptors on their surface, each one capable of receiving a single message. Once the message is received, it is transmitted to the center, or nucleus, of the cell, where it is processed and its order then directed to the specific gene that does the job that is being called for. For this system to work, the right gene has to be found, which means that the gene for this function has to have a fixed location in all cells.

There are estimated to be about one hundred thousand genes, but though very ambitious long-term research is now under way, the locations of only a few of them are known as yet. And, as to their function, even less is known.

Genetics of Breast Cancer

To go back to our computer analogy, we know that you can introduce into a computer "bugs" that give instructions that were not built into the system. In the 1960s and 1970s we learned that there are viruses that can do the same thing in human cells. They can produce genetic instructions that result in stimulated cell growth. Once such viruses infect a cell, the instructions—*viral oncogenes*—override the genes that regulate normal growth and cause rapid, uncontrolled growth.

Sometimes the normal controlling genes, called *cellular oncogenes*, themselves become corrupted. They then come to resemble viral oncogenes and can also stimulate abnormal growth.

The presence of such oncogenes is one of the prerequisites for the conversion of a normal cell to a cancer cell.

Certain viruses that can cause cancer may be defective—that is, they may not carry their own oncogenes. When these viruses infect cells, they fuse with chromosomes next to existing growth-regulating genes and stimulate their otherwise quiet neighbors to become uncontrollably active.

In recent years, a second kind of gene involved in cancer has been identified. Called *suppressor genes*, these normally produce substances that slow or suppress abnormal growth. If they are damaged, cancer begins to appear. This discovery is particularly important because suppressor genes appear to act like an "off switch" and thus may be useful to stop further growth of cancer.

The substances that bind to cell surface receptors to initiate cell growth are called *growth factors*. Abnormal growth factor production may stimulate the growth of cancer cells. Cancer cells can sometimes manufacture their own growth factor and thus empower themselves to reproduce endlessly. And sometimes cancer cells produce receptors that are abnormal and that behave as if they've been stimulated by growth factors though there are none present.

BREAST CANCER GENES

In 1995, BRCA1 and BRCA2, two genes directly related to breast cancer, were cloned. This procedure permits large amounts of purified genetic material to be produced so that the structure and function of each gene can be closely studied. Women with defective BRCA1 genes have an 85 percent risk of getting breast cancer and a 45 percent risk of getting cancer of the ovary by age seventy. Of the five percent of breast cancers attributed each year to genetic causes (see page 243), about half can be explained by BRCA1. At this time we know less about BRCA2, but anticipate that it will account for an additional 20 percent of hereditary breast cancers. There is also evidence that errors in BRCA1 may be found in random (non–heredity-determined) breast cancers. In such patients, normal cells have unaltered BRCA1, while in tumor cells this gene is damaged.

Tests for both the breast cancer genes are becoming widely

available. As a result, more patients who have had breast cancer, and their relatives, will be learning whether they carry an abnormal form of these genes. What to do with this information remains unclear, particularly since each of the genes has already been found to have a large number of possible mutations, some of which appear to have more significance than others. At present there are two options for reducing the risk of breast cancer that may be associated with BRCA1 or BRCA2. The first is to begin early to participate in a screening program that includes annual mammography. The other is to consider prophylactic mastectomies. Ultimately, a preventive treatment is the most desirable alternative, but none is yet available.

Metastasis

Uncontrolled growth is characteristic of cancer cells, but it is not their only property. Cancer cells also have the ability to travel from one part of the body to another—that is, to metastasize. They accomplish this by breaking through the supporting tissue and entering lymphatics or blood vessels.

We are continually learning about the biology of metastasis. One aspect we have discovered is that a cell that will metastasize seems to develop the ability to produce enzymes that digest proteins and enable the cell to invade normal tissue.

There is another group of genes whose role is very different. These genes seem to have the ability to inhibit metastasis. When these genes are inactivated, the cancer can spread.

The Results of Research

If ever there was a time to ask, "What does it all mean?," this is it. From an extremely complex group of findings, we are busy simultaneously trying to understand the cause of cancer and also to treat it. Molecular biologists and biochemists are hard at work on the former task, and from their still incomplete findings, pharmacologists are working to come up with drugs that will save people's lives.

Current research aims to attack uncontrolled cell growth on many fronts:

- by competing with growth factors to attach themselves to receptors or by rendering growth factors inactive
- by interrupting the message of "turned on" receptors before they reach the cell nucleus
- by inactivating abnormal oncogenes or their products
- by introducing new genes to replace abnormal suppressor genes
- by stopping production of the enzymes cancer cells use to invade normal surrounding tissue

One trick that is being worked on is to try to manufacture receptor material to inject into patients. The growth factors would then "make the mistake" of attaching themselves to this injected material before they reached the receptors on the cells themselves.

Still concentrating on receptors, drugs are being developed that would block those on the surface of a cell from accepting cell growth-stimulator chemicals.

Another line of research concentrates on the activity within the cell after the growth factor has reached it. When a particular receptor on the outside of a cell is activated, that sets off a chemical reaction on its other end, the one inside the cell. If you can interfere with this reaction deep in the cell, then growth will not take place. New drugs are being developed to accomplish this.

Poisoning the enemy—so to speak—is still another technique that is already in use. In order for genes to duplicate themselves and cells to divide, a finely tuned orchestration of many genes must take place. One approach is to let cells manufacture genes but to feed them the wrong nutrients—antimetabolite drugs like 5-fluorouracil—so that the new genes are inactive. The trouble with this treatment is that it is only moderately selective and may interfere with gene manufacture in healthy as well as cancerous cells.

We are now looking for drugs that will be "smarter," that will turn off only the specific genes related to uncontrolled growth. Their effects will be so focused that they will be able to pinpoint cancer cells and avoid damaging normal cells.

Growth-suppressor genes are important because their narrowly focused range of activity enables them to turn off growth without harming the cells. In order for cancer to develop, suppressor genes such as retinoblastoma and p53 have to be inactivated. To replace these defective genes by introducing a normal suppressor gene into the cell would require gene transplant, the technique that is now so often discussed. In fact; as of this writing, two children with severe immune-deficiency disease have received experimental gene transplants in therapy at the National Institutes of Health. The treatment worked and the children are now back in school. We are hoping that this technique will be successful and put to use for more people, breast cancer patients included.

As we have seen, cancers rely on certain enzymes not found in normal cells for their ability to digest proteins and thus to slice through tissue and infiltrate. Normal cells do not have the enzymes that do this work. There are chemicals that effectively block these implicated enzymes and they will be tested on human cancers shortly.

Another avenue that is being pursued is to starve out the cancer. The technique that is being investigated is to shut off chemically the growth of the small blood vessels that nourish the tumor. A drug has been tested in animals that is said to do just that. It reportedly has few side effects and will soon be used in trials with cancer patients.

IMMUNOLOGY

Although molecular biology is the field in which the most important advances are being made in cancer research, scientists involved in immunology also have an important role to play. This is true despite the fact that a great deal of work that was done in immunology and cancer in the 1970s turned out to have disappointing results. The drugs that were used to "increase immunity" did not accomplish that goal for various reasons:

• Perhaps immunity does not play as significant a role in cancer as it does in other diseases.

- Immunity may be suppressed by the tumor in ways we don't yet understand.
- While there may be functions of the immune process that do work to suppress cancer growth, there may be others that are actually used by tumors to facilitate such growth.

There are, however, some areas in which progress is being made. In work with what are called biological response modifiers, the goal is to selectively stimulate aspects of the patient's immune system as well as to treat the illness. We have been able to identify substances such as interferon and interleukin 2 that are part of the body's natural immune system. By isolating the genes that manufacture these substances and using genetic engineering techniques, we can then produce them in large quantities.

When these substances have been given to patients, the results have been mixed: interferon has not been found to be useful in the treatment of breast cancer. Though interleukin 2 has been shown to be helpful in treating cancer of the kidney, it has not yet seemed effective for people with breast cancer. There are, however, additional regulators of immunity available, and any one of them, singly or in combination, may prove to be effective against breast cancer.

Progress is also being made in the manufacture of antibodies, proteins that attack specific targets, or antigens, by binding to them. We have known for a long time, for example, about the effectiveness of an antitoxin in preventing tetanus. What we actually do is to give a large dose of the antibody against the poison produced by tetanus bacteria.

Antibodies are part of the natural defenses of all animals, including humans. *Monoclonal antibodies* is the name given to antibodies produced by the progeny of a single cell. These antibodies have the ability to detect one specific chemical on the surface of a cell. Because of this skill, they are able to distinguish between cells that even under a microscope look identical.

An effort is now being made to use monoclonal antibodies against cancer by having them

- isolate targets that are unique to the surface of a cancer cell

- destroy the target on their own, or
- carry a drug or radioactive substance that will destroy it
- bind to receptors on the surface of the cancer cell to prevent the attachment of growth factors

Monoclonal antibody to the protein product of HER2/neu (see page 156), a breast-cancer-associated gene produced by molecular methods and made to resemble a human antibody, is being used with modest success alone and in combination with chemotherapy to treat women with advanced breast cancer.

We are learning that some of the cells, such as *LAK cells* and *T cells*, that are associated with the immune system can be activated and stimulated to attack cancer cells specifically. Relatively few people with breast cancer have received this form of therapy and there is little we can yet say about its effectiveness.

PATIENT STUDIES

We have been talking, up to now, about what is sometimes called bench research—the laboratory bench, that is. Now we will consider what can be learned from studying patients, through clinical research.

How Are Clinical Studies Put Together?

In order to tell whether a drug or a treatment method is effective and safe, it has to be tried on enough people and under circumstances that are well enough controlled to give us reliable evidence. Sometimes you can find these conditions at a single very large institution, but in actuality, most of this work is done by cooperative groups that have been organized specifically to conduct such studies, usually with funding from the National Cancer Institute.

The largest of these groups include the Eastern Cooperative Oncology Group (ECOG), the National Surgical Adjuvant Breast and Bowel Project (NSABP), the Cancer and Leukemia Group B (CALGB), and the Southwestern Oncology Group (SWOG). Each group has many separate medical institutions affiliated with it, and if you decide to participate in a clinical trial it will probably be at one of these institutions.

To begin with, a study must be designed so that all participating researchers use a uniform approach in seeking answers to particular questions about chemotherapy, or surgical treatment, or causes of the disease, or other areas of investigation.

Preliminary planning includes answering questions such as these:

- What is the reason for this investigation?
- Who should be treated?
  Age range
  Sex
  Patient's condition
  Stage of disease
  Previous treatment
- What treatment will be given?
  Specific surgery
  Specific adjuvant treatment
  Drug regimen including combination, dosage,
    frequency, schedule
- How will patients' progress be measured?
- How will information be gathered?
- How will information be analyzed?

If several different treatments are going to be considered, patients are often selected randomly to receive one or another of them. Sometimes, in order to ensure impartial and clear results, a study is designed so that some patients receive the drug that is being tested and others receive a placebo, a substance that has no pharmaceutical effect.

Patients are then treated and carefully followed by means of regular tests and visits. For uniformity and reliability, particularly complex tests may be performed by specially designated laboratories. Records are kept of the specific information the study was designed to gather, and the results are analyzed by study statisticians.

Often, if patients getting a particular treatment do especially well, the study will be stopped so that all patients can be given what has been shown to be the more effective treatment.

The Phases of Drug Testing

When a new drug is being tested, the study is usually conducted in several stages, or phases, to ensure the safest possible conditions for the patients and the most rigorous gathering of information.

PHASE I

- Before any drug is tested on human beings it must be shown, through animal testing, or preclinical testing, to be safe and potentially effective.
- An application is filed with the Food and Drug Administration (FDA) to begin clinical studies, using the drug on human beings.
- The treatment and the possible risks are carefully explained to patients who may wish to participate, and they are informed that they may receive a placebo and not the new drug. Patients also must sign an informed-consent form.
- The plan must be approved by the institutional review board (IRB) of each participating facility.
- Initially, the drug is given to participating patients in low doses.
- Dosages are gradually increased to determine effectiveness, side effects, and toxicity.

Should you join a Phase I drug test? It all depends. If you have already had an unsuccessful course of treatment that you think was as vigorous as possible, you may welcome the chance to try something new. There is certainly reason to believe it may work because, to get to a Phase I study, the drug has to have shown promise in preclinical trials. Only a few drugs a year ever get to this point.

263

On the other hand, a Phase I drug should not be used if you have not yet tried an already established treatment that is known to be effective. The potential side effects that are already known from animal studies should be thoroughly reviewed, and it should be explained to you that there may only be a small chance that the drug will help you.

PHASE II

By the time a drug gets to this point, we already know quite a lot about its potential benefits, side effects, toxicity, and appropriate dose levels. The Phase II study explores the drug's benefits for patients with a particular form of cancer.

- Only the drug being studied is given to participating patients.
- One or more fixed dose levels are administered.

Before you join a Phase II study, you should be assured that there are already data that suggest that it will be helpful in your particular situation. You should be sure there is not an already established treatment that might benefit you, and that potential side effects have been thoroughly explained to you.

PHASE III

A Phase III drug has been shown to have good potential as a treatment for a particular condition. The questions that remain are: Is it better than treatments already in use? How does it measure up against other drugs or combinations of drugs? In order to answer these questions, some patients participating in the study will be given the new treatment and some will be given treatments already in use.

Consider these factors carefully as they relate to your own case, and also bear in mind that when a new treatment is being tested in a Phase III study, you won't necessarily get it, even if you are participating in the study. The selection of patients within the study to receive the new treatment is made on a random basis so that comparisons can be made between established and new therapies. You may turn out to be in a control group that does not receive the new treatment.

Phase III studies are the least problematic for participating patients in the sense that we know a great deal about the treatment, its side effects, proper dosages, et cetera, by the time we get to this point.

The Ethics of Clinical Trials

It used to be that people would say they didn't want to be "guinea pigs," that they wanted to be sure of a drug's effectiveness before they tried it. In recent years, however, many patients who are gravely ill have been eager to try whatever is available and relatively safe, if it shows promise of helping them.

In terms of advances in medical treatment, a great deal of what we know about breast cancer has come from such clinical trials:

It was an NSABP trial that established that lumpectomy and radiation are as effective in treating Stage I and Stage II breast cancer as mastectomy.

A group of researchers at the National Tumor Institute in Milan established that if cancer has spread to the lymph nodes near the breast, using adjuvant CMF chemotherapy after surgery was better at preventing recurrence than no further treatment at all. This set the stage for the broad use of preventive hormone therapy and chemotherapy.

Several groups have demonstrated that even in patients with local breast cancer and negative lymph nodes, chemotherapy can push cure rates up.

In addition to the studies related to basic science research that we have discussed, clinical studies now under way include investigations of

- the length of time patients should be treated with tamoxifen
- new drug combinations for chemotherapy
- drugs that reduce the toxicity of already existing treatments
- the use of chemotherapy for patients whose tumors were one centimeter or less

- the effectiveness of combining hormone therapy and chemotherapy rather than using one method alone
- the possibility that intensive treatment that requires bone-marrow transplant can cure otherwise incurable patients
- the use of chemotherapy to reduce tumors to a size that permits breast-conserving surgery
- the effectiveness of radiation therapy in the treatment of *in situ* cancers

Obviously these studies have great potential value. You should consider participating under the following circumstances:

- Established therapy to help you has been exhausted, *or* the new treatment is likely to produce benefits just as good or better than established therapy.
- You are fully informed about what the study is intended to accomplish.
- You understand why this treatment offers you a special opportunity.
- You have been told the range of possible side effects and have been assured that every effort will be made to limit them.

How Do I Find Out About Clinical Trials?

If you have decided that you want to look into the possibility of participating in a clinical trial, there are several ways you can proceed:

- Start by talking to your physician. Many breast cancer specialists have trained at cancer research centers and regularly participate in their clinical studies.
- Research centers around the country enlist the help of local physicians. Your doctor may be taking part in a study by one of these centers or she may be able to refer you to someone else who is.

266

- You can call 1-800-4-CANCER, the Cancer Information Service of the National Cancer Institute. This phone number gives you access to PDQ, a computer service that will produce a printout of all ongoing breast cancer trials, with the names and phone numbers of the principal investigators.
- NABCO, the National Alliance of Breast Cancer Organizations (212-719-0154), can also refer you to sources of information about clinical trials.

Consensus Conferences

Despite all the studies and analyses, serious questions sometimes remain as to how to proceed in the treatment of cancer. The National Cancer Institute has tried to deal with such thorny questions by calling Consensus Conferences of clinical investigators, supporting professionals, and patients.

Their purpose is to evaluate available scientific information, to resolve safety and effectiveness issues, to advance the understanding of technology or of a medical question, and then to provide information that will be helpful to health professionals and to the public. In practical terms, these conferences are a way of consolidating what we know and of recommending what ought to be done in day-to-day practice.

The conferences have helped crystallize certain treatment standards, they have aroused useful debate, and they have stimulated research and analysis that may prove useful in finding the cause of and the cure for breast cancer.

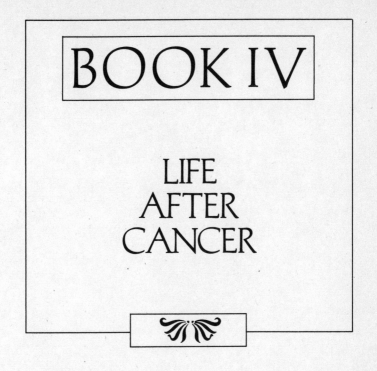

BOOK IV

LIFE
AFTER
CANCER

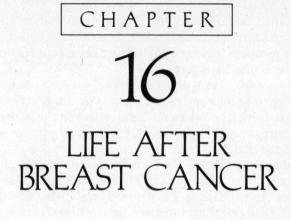

CHAPTER

16

LIFE AFTER
BREAST CANCER

☙❧

Thre is no particular program for coping emotionally with breast cancer, no regimen that I, as a doctor, can prescribe with assurances to you that, taken twice daily, you'll be all right. This chapter, therefore, relies heavily not on advice but on the experiences of the women I've known and heard about who have had this illness.

No sane person would choose to have breast cancer or, having had it, would say that it was an ennobling experience. Nobody who has had a grave illness, or who has lived through the experience of surgery, or who has worried about the effects of powerful treatments, would mouth such platitudes.

One of my patients whose breast cancer was only one of a series of terrible life events described a time she completely lost her temper when a self-avowed "religious" neighbor advised her,

"Be thankful, dear. God doesn't give us more than we can bear."

And yet, difficult though it is to live through, many patients who have recovered say that having had breast cancer does eventually recede into their past.

One woman, seven years after her surgery, said, "I think about it when I go for my yearly mammogram, and I sometimes scare myself when I read about recurrences in the paper, but it's just not part of my daily agenda anymore. Life goes on, the good stuff and the bad."

Another woman said, "I remember that when I found out, my first reaction was, 'Oh, my God, I'll lose my breast!' Then I realized that wasn't the issue. I was afraid I would die, and because I couldn't talk about that, I focused on my breast. Later on, each treatment made me feel safer, and—believe it or not—I was afraid to stop chemotherapy. Now, every year that goes by, I worry a little less."

That is not to say that this is by any means a trivial matter or that it does not leave its mark on you, as these two women report: "I've become much more of a health nut than I ever was before. I listen to my body more . . . sometimes I even feel I'm being a little hypochondriac. But the good side is, I read a lot about taking care of yourself and I watch my diet more—hardly any fats at all— and I'm religious about going for physicals and mammograms right on schedule."

"I can go for months feeling great and I don't even think about cancer. Even though I see my mastectomy scar every day, I've just gotten used to it and it doesn't make any difference. But the week I have to see my doctor, I'm a wreck. I never can figure out what the problem is until the visit is over and he tells me I'm okay."

The period after surgery, just after they have come home from the hospital, is the time when most women experience their highest level of depression and anxiety. There has been an enormous amount to get through from the time they first realized something was wrong, through the period of evaluating their choices and making decisions, through the surgery itself. Now they must face picking up their lives again and also coping with whatever further treatment has been decided upon.

"When I first got out of the hospital, I was afraid I wasn't going to be able to manage everything that was waiting for me. You know, even though you wish the nurses wouldn't wake you at six in the morning to take your temperature, and the residents wouldn't keep asking you the same questions over and over again, still those are signs you're being taken care of. You get a little infantilized in the hospital, as if you don't have to take care of yourself, you have all these nursemaids to do it. And then— boom! You're home and people expect you to be a responsible grown-up again."

Women have various ways of dealing with the issues of self-image, relationships, career, and continued treatment after they have had breast cancer. One woman said, "I've always got a list for everything—food shopping, my kids' schedules, what I want to tell my boss the next time I accidentally-on-purpose meet him at the coffee shop. After my breast surgery there were so many things to worry about, I decided to make a list. It had some pretty ridiculous items like: '1. Afraid to walk the dog. Maybe he'll hurt my arm,' followed by '2. Hire a dog-walker for a few weeks.' It sounds sappy but I even had on there when I thought my husband and I could start having sex again. Just putting it there gave me the sense that everything has a chance of falling into place if I cross each item off one at a time."

The unknowns that women face after breast cancer lie in many corners of their lives, and some of them, as we'll see in the following pages, quite naturally cause a great deal of concern. But after a while, when the "tincture of time" has had a chance to do its work, there seems to be a universal ebbing of anxiety:

"The first few weeks, that's all I could think about—my cancer, my mastectomy, my reconstruction. It's as if I had to give all my energy to that. I was pretty depressed, I guess, but then those dark periods would alternate with normal times, when I'd be laughing with my kids and getting it all together. Gradually, there were more good times than bad."

GETTING THROUGH THE CRISIS

Where Does Help Come From?

Though there are variations in their reactions, most women who have breast cancer go through the crisis without long-lasting psychological or sexual problems. Some of them use short-term professional therapy to help them manage, but many accomplish this by becoming actively involved in their treatment, as well as by accepting the support of family and friends and other women who have had breast cancer. They also find groups such as Reach to Recovery, Cancer Care, the nurses or social service workers at the hospital, the American Cancer Society, and other individuals and organizations in the community of great practical as well as emotional support.

Very often, not only you, but also your life partner and other family members can avail themselves of such services. It may be helpful to remember that you're not the only novice in this game. So are your family and friends. They are often frightened for you and for themselves and they may be worried about whether they'll be able to give you the care you need. They may not know what to say or how to say it. Particularly during the sometimes long haul of extended chemotherapy, when you may need more help than usual, children can forget why their mother is not as available to them as she ordinarily is.

One woman who was suffering from nausea during her chemotherapy said, "I don't know why, but washing out the bathtub made me feel sick. It became a real issue with my sixteen-year-old son, your typical teenage slob. Eventually, I explained to him that—irrational or not—this was a time in our lives when he was going to have to go more than halfway. He did try harder after that and, luckily, my medication was changed and I didn't have the problem anymore."

Another woman, in speaking of her friends' concern, said, "Sometimes the sympathy of my friends and family was a burden for me. Everyone was so sad. I could see how worried they were and, in a way, it scared me even more. I used to enjoy being with people once in a while who didn't know about my cancer, so I could forget about it myself for a couple of hours. But those feelings weren't really important. In spite of a twinge like that once in a while, what kept me going was the support I got from the people around me."

That last is the recurring theme from women who have had breast cancer: being able to accept the support and practical help of friends and family is what got them through.

To become seriously ill, whatever the disease, often carries with it an element of shame or guilt that is irrational but no less real. There is a part of us that believes that being less than the picture of radiant health portrayed everywhere around us means that we've somehow failed as human beings, that we're inadequate. As an extension of that attitude, some women seem to feel that they have let their husbands down by getting breast cancer.

One woman expressed those feelings on a recent television report on breast cancer. Asked whether she was upset about losing her breast, she said something like, "I guess I don't mind so much, but I feel bad for my husband."

Her husband, without missing a beat, replied, "I don't care about that. You and me and the kids, we're a family. That's the important thing."

What was impressive about this man was not only his loyalty but also his ability to express it. That, for all concerned, seems to be of primary importance. Being able to talk about your illness is key to your well-being. In general, I have found that it is not psychiatrists who seem to be of the most help in this instance, but other women. They may have been trained in counseling, as social workers, nurses, or physical therapists, or they may not be in the helping professions at all. Women who have had breast cancer can often be especially useful to those who now have the illness, both in terms of practical advice based on their experience and as a source of emotional support.

Women who have recovered say they frequently get telephone calls from "friends of friends" who have heard they had breast cancer and want advice. "I feel like there's a powerful underground network of women helping each other," one of them said.

One patient who had recently learned she had breast cancer said, "People I never knew had breast cancer are just coming out of the woodwork. It almost seems like every other person I know has had it, or her sister did. And most of them want to help."

Group sessions led by a woman experienced in counseling can be helpful, as can counselors with special experience with the issues of breast cancer. I work with one counselor who is so good that I consider her my greatest resource. She'll talk to women any time, even on the telephone before formally meeting them. It's not only her professional training that makes her so good, but also the fact that she has had mastectomies and chemotherapy herself.

Her view is that "women need short-term support to take

them through what they have to do and then they have to go on with their lives." She's right. Cancer doesn't make your life better, but it shouldn't take it over.

How Do I Handle My Job?

Let's begin this section with the good news and then go back to the practical questions and the strategies that seem to have succeeded best in this crucial area of breast cancer's impact on a job or a career. The first thing to be said is that having had breast cancer and then returned to work has not had a negative long-term impact on the careers of most women. That is not to say that there are no problems. As we will discuss, there are practical considerations like insurance coverage, getting time off for adjuvant treatment, and the physical demands of the job. There are also more abstract questions that have to do with the attitude of coworkers and of company executives toward your illness and their perception of your ability to do the job well.

HEALTH INSURANCE

"I'm pretty new on this job and I'm afraid they'll be so mad about these medical bills I'm submitting to the insurance company, I may be fired."

This not-uncommon worry has a straightforward answer: you can't be fired for being sick. Your health insurance can't be terminated if you get cancer, as long as you're able to do your job. The information you or your doctor provides in connection with an insurance claim is confidential. If you do leave your job, you are entitled to coverage at a group rate for a period of time until you can make other arrangements.

Unfortunately—and surely society must very quickly address the problem that over thirty-five million Americans do not have health insurance—these new insurance arrangements can be very hard to make and also very expensive. Insurers often make it difficult for people who have "expensive" illnesses to get new coverage, especially when they are applying on their own and not as part of a group. Even in group coverage, there may be excessive waiting periods before the costs of treatment for a preexisting illness are reimbursed. If you are concerned about your

276

insurance coverage you should consult the hospital social worker. These professionals are often very knowledgeable and can refer you to specialists in the field of health insurance or give you advice themselves. There are, for example, professional and social organizations throughout the country that offer health insurance to their membership and that accept new members quite readily. In many instances, there is an open period once a year, a time when unaffiliated people can apply to health insurance companies and be accepted without meeting the usual eligibility requirements. Again, however, the coverage that is offered may be expensive.

If you are employed at the time of your illness and are covered by your company's medical insurance policy, it probably makes sense to stay at your job, at least for the period that you are receiving treatment. I have seen some patients and their families beside themselves with worry about health insurance. (It probably makes sense to stay on your job for other reasons, too. You are undergoing enough difficulties at the moment, without adding another stressful change.)

WHOM SHOULD I TELL AT WORK?

The question of how open you are going to be about your illness, especially at work, is an extremely personal one. Some women talk freely about having breast cancer and seem not to suffer any unpleasant consequences. Others have what appear to be legitimate reasons for not wishing their private affairs to become public, particularly in the workplace. They may have a very strong sense of privacy. They don't even want the word *cancer* to be written on their health insurance forms lest other people find out about it. (This is not possible. The diagnosis must be noted in order for you to receive insurance benefits and any disability pay.)

Such women don't want to "cope with their coworkers" in the sense of having to talk about their treatment and other aspects of their illness. They may also worry that their careers will suffer: "I'm in a really competitive field. One word of my having the Big C and I'm right off the fast track."

You may indeed be in a work situation where it is simply not a good idea to discuss the details of your illness. There are certain

277

highly competitive or cutthroat businesses and professions where the "fast track" doesn't make accommodation for serious illness. In those situations, taking time off—and being discreet about what was wrong—may serve you best. It is worth repeating that filing an insurance claim does not automatically trigger disclosure of what is wrong with you. In most situations, the insurer and the company's benefits department are specifically enjoined from such disclosure. Many companies also have a system under which you can send your claim directly to the insurer.

A problem sometimes arises for women on jobs that require a lot of physical effort. They usually can manage sick time for their illness but they are concerned that if word gets around that they had cancer, their employers and coworkers will incorrectly conclude that they'll never again be able to work hard. They are particularly worried that they may not get time off for adjuvant radiation or systemic therapy or that they may be fatigued after those treatments. In these situations, it may be best to figure out who among your supervisors is likely to be the most sympathetic. Take that person into your confidence and ask him or her to help you devise a plan that will work best for the company and for you. If you are a member of a union, talk to the shop steward or some other union official about what benefits and time off you can expect.

But . . . there is no reason to assume that people will act badly. As we have seen, the breast cancer rates in this country are unfortunately high enough that the majority of your colleagues will have people close to them who have had the illness. Furthermore, enough well-known women—Betty Ford and Nancy Reagan among them—have made no secret of their breast cancer and have helped those who don't have personal experience with the disease to understand it.

As a result, most people will react helpfully and sympathetically, as this woman describes: "I talked to the head of our personnel department when I first found out about my cancer. She told me that she'd be of whatever help she could, but she also went out of her way to drop some remark like, 'Of course, none of us have any way of knowing what's on your medical claims.'"

However, the most important point here is that even if the information becomes known—either because you yourself talk about it or by some other means—it does not seem to have long-term detrimental effects on the careers of most people. Whatever its initial impact in the workplace, once the original crisis of the illness is over, any shock to your colleagues your cancer has caused seems to wear off.

That also seems to work out when, eventually, women do make job changes (and this seems to be true of both women and men, whether they have had breast cancer or other cancers). People forget. They see what you are doing in your career today and many of them assume that "what's past is past."

That obviously is not true in every case. There are some stories about women who were passed over, particularly for a new job, because of their illness. Nevertheless, if a potential new employer does know you have had cancer, there is no point in denying it. There are laws in most states against discrimination in hiring and you may want to avail yourself of them.

It is an unfortunate reality that a certain number of misguided conceptions and unsympathetic attitudes about cancer are out there in the workplace. They are cruel and ignorant and we should be doing everything we can to eliminate them. In fact, as noted, most states and localities have legislation on their books against overt discrimination and you should utilize the law's protection in the unlikely case that it may become necessary. (See page 300 for a free booklet on such issues.)

Fortunately, that kind of drastic action is rarely necessary. Many women with breast cancer report that they shared with their colleagues everything that was going on and that they had no reason to regret that course of action. Though there may have been some awkwardness on the job when they first became sick, after a while, when they were back at work, most people seemed to forget about the problem.

How Do I Handle My Personal Life?

SEXUALITY

We talked earlier in the book about how important the breast is to many women and men as a symbol of sexuality. After breast surgery, couples need to work out their private lives, striking a balance between rushing back into sexual relations to "prove" everything is the same as ever, as against allowing unspoken fears and inhibitions to build up and make it difficult to resume a fulfilling physical relationship. The old signals may not serve: the husband may have doubts about whether his wife is ready for lovemaking and she may mistake this for aversion. Or the woman who has had breast surgery may feel quite fragile and need time to slowly reaccustom herself to making love.

One woman described an even more subtle problem: "In our relationship, when one or the other of us is in some trouble, we tend to cuddle a lot and get comfort from being physically close. That often leads to sex—except now I'm just ready for the cuddling and not the next step. I need some time to get used to my body again."

We have learned over the years how important it is in a good physical relationship for partners to tell each other what they need and want. This is especially important now, after breast cancer.

One patient had a funny revelation when she talked to her long-time lover about how worried she was about her appearance. She said, "When I was a girl, we walked around with a tape measure to keep checking that our dimensions were right, and girls went through all sorts of agony, especially if their chest wasn't big enough. Well, after my mastectomy, mine sure wasn't, but when I said something like that to Jim, he looked at me as if I was crazy. 'Listen, I've always loved the way you looked because you're so elegantly slim—like a model or one of those Twenties pictures of some woman golf star.' "

After breast cancer, single women who are seeking a new relationship may worry about how a new person will react and they may be reluctant to mention their illness: "I'm not dating anyone now, and I'm afraid that if this gets around, I'm doomed to spending my life alone."

However, as discussed several times earlier in the book, the good stories seem to be at least as numerous as the bad. A forty-year-old patient told of meeting the "man of her dreams" only about six weeks after breast surgery: "All the time we were getting to know each other, I was thinking either 'Why didn't this happen last year?' or else 'Why couldn't this happen next year, when the scars will look better?' "

Certainly, for most women, the best course of action seems to be to give yourself time after the surgery to make peace with all you have been experiencing before beginning a new relationship. But this same woman said, "Rushing into a relationship with

LIFE AFTER BREAST CANCER

Fred at that point in my life was probably foolhardy. But it turned out to be the best psychological medicine I could take. It made me feel that I was still a desirable woman."

Not every story of a new relationship turns out so well. Some people may shy away from what they see as the added responsibility of becoming involved with someone who has been ill. They may have fears about illness in general. Obviously, you won't want to share the facts of your illness with everyone you meet, but as you become close to new people, you will probably find it most comfortable to tell them about what is, after all, a major event in your life.

A new attitude has been emerging lately: young women especially have been writing and saying that they don't want to go "into the closet" about breast cancer. They are proud of their bodies, breast cancer or no; they want to be able to talk about their experiences as women, including their illnesses, without the shame that women commonly used to feel about their physical lives: about menstruation, or the details of childbirth—or breast cancer.

FAMILY AND FRIENDS

"My marriage wasn't that strong before all this happened. I just don't think it will survive so much trouble, but I'm in no condition right now to take on another big upheaval."

"It's so strange, we used to have a lot of rocky times before, but it feels like this breast cancer thing has brought us closer together. I think when you have hard times, both people come to realize how much you rely on each other."

There seems to be a surprisingly low incidence of divorce among my patients. Perhaps that is due to a reordering of priorities; perhaps both partners are unlikely to make changes during a stressful time; perhaps having been through such a crisis together strengthens the relationship thereafter. Though everyone has heard or read about husbands and lovers who do not come through in a crisis, the overwhelming majority of them do. And, whether married or single, heterosexual or homosexual, women who have had rewarding social and sexual lives before their breast cancer seem to take up where they left off and build those good lives again.

The need for honesty with your husband or partner is pretty straightforward, but it is also important to be forthcoming with your children. Even young children need to be told why you are going to the hospital or for treatment, and they also need to have some idea of what's going on with your body. There's a good analogy between frankness about this and giving your kids information about sex. You tell them as much as they can understand and absorb, without overwhelming them, or being evasive, or making them think there's some terrible secret.

One man, whose wife was ill with breast cancer when their daughters were twelve and fourteen, said that one of the girls, who is now twenty, recently expressed great anger that she had been neglected during the illness, that no one in the family had seemed to care about what was happening to her and her sister. Her father said, "But, Joan, your mother was really sick. We had to put all our effort into taking care of her." And Joan replied, "You should have tried. We could have died or something, too, and nobody would have noticed."

The problem is painful and complex. To say that more communication was probably needed is much too facile a comment. When you are gravely ill you put all your energy into fighting the illness. To also be an especially sensitive and participating parent at this time is extremely difficult. Even so, it would be helpful if the parent who is not ill would bear in mind that the children may be frightened or even angry at what is happening to their mother and to their normal family life. Talking about the course of treatment and what their mother will be doing and feeling can alleviate some, if not all, of their anxieties.

Dealing with older children, especially girls and young women, may be harder, since they may very well fear that what has happened to you is going to happen to them. Refer them to the chapter in this book on risk factors. Explain that the information we have is statistical. It does not mean that they are doomed to develop breast cancer. If one of the doctors who have taken care of you is particularly compassionate and helpful, ask your daughter if she would like to talk to him.

IN SOCIAL SITUATIONS

After surgery, when they are busy working on reestablishing their own identity, some women choose to "stay private" because they don't want to concern themselves with other people's reactions. They want to do their own adjusting before they cope with others. One woman said, "I don't want people looking at my chest trying to figure out which breast I lost and then my having to make them feel less embarrassed when I catch them at it."

Other women seem to have a great need to talk about it, to discuss what they were learning about their illness as well as the emotional impact of the disease:

"It felt good for me to air my feelings. I called my friends and family right away and people really rallied round. I needed to talk about it a lot and to get a lot of feedback. It gave me confidence that people cared about me and that was important, especially right before I went into surgery."

"I couldn't bring myself to cook the first day or two after every chemotherapy treatment. One of my friends kept track of when I had to go and she'd bring some tasty little meal over to tempt me. Am I glad she was in on what was going on!"

These women and many others like them were able to accept help and support from the community around them. They gained a great deal from being able to let other people know about their illness.

Above all, women say that they do not want to be pitied: "I'm used to being the one who helps other people and I take pretty good care of my own affairs besides. I almost wish I'd kept my mouth shut about this because now I can't stand it when people are so obvious about feeling sorry for me."

If you have friends who are so ignorant as to think they'll catch breast cancer from you or so unfeeling as to let your illness make a difference in your relationship—well, they were not friends worth having. Most women with breast cancer say that their family and friends were so helpful and sympathetic that they could not have come through without them. They also tell stories of the occasional individual who could not seem to cope with their troubles. "Fair-weather friends," they used to be called, and no great loss.

THE ELDERLY

"My forty-five-year-old son talks to the doctor as if I'm not in the room. Does he think having breast cancer has affected my IQ?

283

The other day he even asked the doctor, right in front of me, 'Is she going to die?'"

Older people who have any serious illness often feel that they are being treated condescendingly or that they are being by-passed when the time arises to make care and treatment decisions. That does, in fact, sometimes happen. Recently, a doctor friend and his wife were outraged that his mother-in-law consulted with a surgeon and oncologist "on her own" and made a decision to have a lumpectomy and radiation therapy against their wishes. My friend was equally annoyed that his mother-in-law's physician did not call to tell him what was going on. He might have been talking about a teenager and not a seventy-six-year-old woman who is still a practicing attorney, albeit one with breast cancer.

Unless a person's age has rendered her mentally incompetent—not a common event—she deserves the same right of self-determination as anyone else. That does not mean that you should not ask for help if you need it. If you are of advanced age and have worked hard to maintain your independence, it can seem a terrible defeat to admit that, at least for a few weeks, you are going to have to stay with someone, or else arrange for someone to come to your home to be with you for a while after breast surgery.

One woman expressed it well. She said, "I've had to face up to the fact that by the time you're my age—I'm eighty-one—not only is your energy level way down, but you don't have quite the same capacity to cope with troubles. I guess it's that you've had your share by this point in your life. So, even though having a mastectomy isn't the big deal for me it would have been when I was younger, I still need a helping hand—and I asked my children for it."

You should get all the help you need, and if it is necessary you should ask for it, either of family and friends, or of the social services available to you. On the other hand, your family should not take the authority for your care away from you as if you were a minor child. Too often, in their effort to "protect" you, your friends and family may talk to your doctors in your place or make arrangements for your care that may not suit you. This kind of behavior can damage your relationship with your doctors and make you feel distrustful of what you are being told.

Most elderly Americans use Medicare as their primary health insurance. You may find that the government reimbursement for the various treatments you must undergo for breast cancer is far less than the actual fees you are being asked to pay. If you do not have supplemental health insurance, you should discuss the matter of payment with the staff of each doctor and facility you are dealing with so that anxiety about bills is not added to the strain of your illness. This is one more place in this book where it is unfortunately necessary to say that our society must quickly turn its attention to ensuring excellent health care for all its citizens. Affordable medical care for the elderly should be an important priority.

Dealing With a High-Risk Cancer

Though you may be in a situation where you have had a recurrence or perhaps extensive metastases, you can still help yourself by making a determined effort to get the very best available treatment.

That, most definitely, does not mean that your life has to be devoted to breast cancer. As we have seen, even women with advanced-stage cancer can, with vigorous treatment, live a long time. Think of yourself as having a chronic illness. Take good care of yourself. Be diligent in going for your examinations and treatment. But leave your disease in the doctor's office. That's the proper place for it.

There are examples every day of women who have done this. One patient, for example, had a very important position in the board of education of a large city school system. She came to my office with a widespread cancer and very little hope. Yet, after a year of chemotherapy, she was so much better that before scheduling her next appointment, she'd take out her calendar to see if she "could squeeze me in." This woman went on to have a rewarding career for many years after her initial grave diagnosis.

This is not a question of denial, of refusing to admit that you are ill. It is a practical acknowledgment that women with breast cancer are living much longer than what used to be considered their "expected time" and are living full and productive lives.

Can I Get Anything Positive Out of This Experience?

The fact is, many women do. A patient who is an actress always felt that being young and beautiful was crucial to her career. She's had a mastectomy and a reconstruction and is still young and beautiful, but she said, "Now I look forward to getting older. Every year that passes since I had cancer is a year gained, not lost."

Having had cancer can be, for some people, a powerful incentive to reorder their priorities. One woman who had breast surgery two years ago said, "I don't sweat the small stuff so much anymore. I used to be a total workaholic on my job and a compulsive neatness freak at home. I still enjoy working and I still like things to be orderly, but I'm more likely to spend Saturday in the park with my pals now and worry about what's in my briefcase some other time."

Many patients seem to have an understanding of the uncertainty of life that people who have not had cancer may not have. A woman who had a mastectomy when her baby was only six months old kept saying, "I only hope I live long enough to bring her up." Well, it's twenty-three years later and that patient is now a grandmother, babysitting for her grandchild.

It would obviously be dishonest to say that every recurrence of breast cancer has so happy an ending. And, in a larger sense, none of us knows with any certainty what life will bring. But I see in many of my patients a special appreciation of family and friends, as well as new gusto for the pleasures of life. Some of them seem to have a renewed religious feeling. Some become active in trying to help other people or in working on the medical and social issues they came to understand through their own illness.

Everyone reacts differently to trouble. There is no "correct" way to cope with or get over an experience as trying as breast cancer. But from what I have observed, women are, in fact, coming through it with intelligence, sensitivity, and a very moving gallantry.

17

THE
SOCIAL ISSUES
OF BREAST CANCER

If, as we have learned, one out of nine women in America will develop breast cancer during her lifetime, why aren't we doing more about it? Why isn't this a primary national concern? Why isn't more effort and more money being put into the problem?

RESEARCH

Breast cancer is now reported as striking 184,000 women a year. That figure, however, does not include the additional twenty percent a year who have preinvasive (*in situ*) cancers but who are not part of these statistics.

287

More than 46,000 women died of breast cancer in 1995.

Though the incidence of breast cancer is slowly rising, the number of people who die of the disease has remained the same over the last several years. In effect, that means that we have a stable number of deaths in a much larger number of cases—proof that we are learning how to treat the disease more effectively. In fact, in 1995, the first significant reduction in the death rate for breast cancer was reported by the National Cancer Institute.

After years of stagnation, the United States government's breast cancer research budget has recently expanded. Funding for basic research into breast cancer's causes, and clinical research directed to finding optimal treatments, have increased and are beginning to be meaningfully supplemented by efforts to investigate risk, prevention, and the impact of breast cancer on the quality of lives of breast cancer survivors and their families.

Current research projects that may offer long-awaited answers include a large study of women's health that is investigating dietary and hormonal links to breast cancer, as well as the Breast Cancer Prevention Trial, which is testing the ability of the drug tamoxifen to prevent the onset of breast cancer in women at high risk (see page 251).

The possible role of environmental exposure to cancer-producing agents is an area of research beginning to attract scientific interest and funding. One ongoing study centers on Long Island, a high-incidence area east of New York City. Among the wide range of causative factors being considered is a possible link between breast cancer and insecticide residues that may have entered the food chain and water supply.

In 1990 the government's breast cancer research budget at the National Cancer Institute (NCI) was $77 million. Since that time, a grass-roots movement of breast-cancer-survivors-turned-advocates has raised the consciousness of congressional leaders, resulting in larger and more diverse research appropriations for breast cancer. In 1995 the NCI's breast cancer research budget was $350 million, and a new program, led by the Department of the Army, was appropriated another $160 million for breast research.

Despite these promising increases, many feel that cancer research in general, and breast cancer research in particular, remain underfunded, and that for more rapid progress we need a shift in spending priorities. To keep this matter in perspective, we should point out that one Stealth bomber costs $865 million. The seventy-five new Stealth bombers the Defense Department wanted in 1991 cost $29 billion. For the fiscal year beginning October 1, 1995, the military budget of the United States government was $266 billion.

DIAGNOSIS AND TREATMENT

Mammograms cost from fifty to two hundred dollars a year, depending largely on the part of the country. (The U.S. average in 1990 was $103. The Middle Atlantic states, with New York in the forefront, are the most expensive for medical treatment.) Of the women most vulnerable to breast cancer—those over forty—only sixty-five percent have had any mammograms in their lifetime and only seventeen percent had one the previous year. Medicare pays fifty-five dollars each, but only for mammograms every *second* year for women over sixty-five. Many insurance policies still do not cover screening mammography, and when government or private insurers are trying to cut costs, it is mammograms they seem to cut first.

Tamoxifen costs about eighty to one hundred dollars a month. Only those women with pharmaceutical insurance are covered for this cost. Women on Medicare must pay for it themselves, as must most other patients. The same is true of any other chemotherapy medication that is taken by mouth.

The cost of sixty Cytoxan tablets, a typical month's supply, was about nineteen dollars a month in 1970. Today, the monthly cost is about $180.

A course of chemotherapy costs anywhere from five thousand to twelve thousand dollars.

A course of radiation therapy after lumpectomy costs seven to twenty-five thousand dollars.

The average cost of a modified radical mastectomy is anywhere from three to eight thousand dollars, depending on where in the country it is performed. Medicare pays about thirteen hundred dollars for the procedure and is expected to pay less in the near future.

Breast reconstruction after mastectomy, a procedure that many women consider essential for their general well-being, costs from about six thousand to about fifteen thousand dollars, depending on which procedure is performed and also on the part of the country. Medicare pays three thousand dollars; many private insurance companies do not pay for the more complicated operations.

THE CONSEQUENCES

There are a lot more numbers like these available. What are the practical results when we add these figures up? Simply put, we are not adequately dealing with an important national crisis. We are not doing enough to find out how to prevent the disease or how to treat it.

People talk so much about "reordering our national priorities" that the phrase has come to seem a cliché, and one that could have a divisive national impact. Who would want to decide that we should, for example, cut back on funds for heart research when so many of our people die of cardiac problems? Or that we should take the $1.1 billion allocated for AIDS research in 1990 and funnel those monies into breast cancer research? Surely we have to do everything we can to fight an epidemic like AIDS, which has destroyed so many thousands of lives so quickly and so terribly.

But the women who suffer from breast cancer need help. They need it also, not instead of. Watching the response to the AIDS epidemic, they were inspired to form their own national movement to eradicate breast cancer through increased research, improved access to care, and extended involvement in decision making. Breast cancer advocates have not argued that current medical research is misplaced—rather, that AIDS and breast cancer, as well as other health concerns, should have higher government priorities for funding than, for example, space and even some defense programs. As Representative Mary Rose Oskar of Ohio said, "We shouldn't be pitting breast cancer against AIDS. We should be pitting it against Star Wars."

The National Breast Cancer Coalition, an organization headquartered in Washington, D.C., has been particularly effective in articulating the need for public action. Also important have been the efforts of the New York–based National Alliance of Breast Cancer Organizations (NABCO) in mounting national educational and direct service programs, and the Susan G. Komen Foundation in Dallas, which has become a major nongovernment source of breast cancer research funding.

In June 1991 a bipartisan coalition of senators and representatives responded to the newly formed breast cancer advocacy movement with a "Breast Cancer Challenge." They called upon the National Cancer Institute and the medical community to join in the fight so that by the year 2000 we will

- understand the causes and find a cure for breast cancer
- reduce the incidence of breast cancer
- reduce the breast cancer mortality rate by fifty percent
- ensure that all women over forty get regular mammograms
- ensure that all mammograms are of the highest quality

As we complete the second edition of this book, where do we stand on meeting these goals? Breast cancer's causes are under intense investigation. Recent advances in genetics are offering important new directions to this research. Both existing and new treatments for breast cancer have continued to improve survival, and new drugs to manage treatment side effects are making it possible for many women to continue their normal work and home lives while they are in treatment.

The incidence of breast cancer has not declined, but more women than ever before are aware of their risk and the importance of following an early detection screening plan: breast self-examination, annual examinations by a physician, and regular mammograms. The government program that offers free breast and cervical screening to underserved women now operates in every state. This has helped to increase the proportion of women over forty who get regular mammograms, but we still have not reached all women who should be screened.

Ensuring that mammograms are of the highest quality is an area where solid progress has been made. The Mammography Quality Standards Act, passed in 1992, has led the Food and

Drug Administration to create a program that assures that all facilities performing mammograms meet federal standards for quality (see page 58).

As gratifying as this progress has been, we have a long way to go before the fight against breast cancer is fully won. We need the same determination that has taken us this far if we are finally to eradicate this terrible disease. Congresswoman Pat Schroeder of Colorado has said, "We have in America all the ingredients needed to beat breast cancer: political will, grass-roots activism, and the medical brainpower."

The question is whether we have the commitment. Certainly women have it—those vast numbers of women who have had breast cancer or who have faced its prospect, or whose close friends or relatives have had it. And if we add to that number the men whose wives and sisters and girlfriends and mothers have had the disease—and those of us who are physicians working with those women—this means that a very large proportion of our people have a stake in a national determination to beat breast cancer.

Whether we can mobilize to achieve this goal remains to be seen.

RESOURCES

NCI CANCER CENTERS

The National Cancer Institute (NCI) supports a number of cancer centers throughout the country that develop and investigate new methods of cancer diagnosis and treatment. Information about referral procedures, treatment costs, and services available to patients can be obtained from the individual cancer centers listed below.

ALABAMA
University of Alabama at Birmingham Comprehensive Cancer Center
Basic Health Sciences
  Building, Room 108
1918 University Boulevard
Birmingham, AL 35294
(205) 934–6612

ARIZONA
University of Arizona Cancer Center
1501 North Campbell Avenue
Tucson, AZ 85724
(602) 626–6372

CALIFORNIA
The Kenneth Norris Jr. Comprehensive Cancer Center
University of Southern
  California
1441 Eastlake Avenue
Los Angeles, CA 90033-0804
(213) 226–2370

Jonsson Comprehensive Cancer Center
University of California at Los
  Angeles
200 Medical Plaza
Los Angeles, CA 90027
(213) 206–0278

City of Hope National Medical Center
Beckman Research Institute
1500 East Duarte Road
Duarte, CA 91010
(818) 359–8111, ext. 2292

University of California at San Diego Cancer Center
225 Dickinson Street
San Diego, CA 92103
(619) 543–6178

COLORADO
University of Colorado Cancer Center
4200 East 9th Avenue, Box B190
Denver, CO 80262
(303) 270–7235

RESOURCES

CONNECTICUT
**Yale University Comprehensive
Cancer Center**
333 Cedar Street
P.O. Box 3333
New Haven, CT 06510
(203) 785–6338

DISTRICT OF COLUMBIA
**Lombardi Cancer Research
Center**
Georgetown University
    Medical Center
3800 Reservoir Road, NW
Washington, DC 20007
(202) 687–2192

FLORIDA
**Sylvester Comprehensive
Cancer Center**
University of Miami Medical
    School
1475 Northwest 12th Avenue
Miami, FL 33136
(305) 548–4800

ILLINOIS
Illinois Cancer Center
17th Floor
200 South Michigan Avenue
Chicago, IL 60604
(312) 986–9980

**University of Chicago Cancer
Research Center**
5841 South Maryland Avenue
Chicago, IL 60637
(312) 702–9200

MARYLAND
**The Johns Hopkins Oncology
Center**
600 North Wolfe Street
Baltimore, MD 21205
(301) 955–8638

MASSACHUSETTS
Dana-Farber Cancer Institute
44 Binney Street
Boston, MA 02115
(617) 732–3214

MICHIGAN
**Meyer L. Prentis
Comprehensive Cancer
Center of Metropolitan
Detroit**
110 East Warren Avenue
Detroit, MI 48201
(313) 745–4329

**University of Michigan Cancer
Center**
101 Simpson Drive
Ann Arbor, MI 48109-0752
(313) 936–9583

MINNESOTA
**Mayo Comprehensive Cancer
Center**
200 First Street Southwest
Rochester, MN 55905
(507) 284–3413

NEW HAMPSHIRE
**Norris Cotton Cancer
Center**
Dartmouth-Hitchcock
    Medical Center
1 Medical Center Drive
Lebanon, NH 03756
(603) 650–5000

NEW YORK
**Memorial Sloan-Kettering
Cancer Center**
1275 York Avenue
New York, NY 10021
1–800–525–2225

**Columbia University
Comprehensive Cancer Center**
College of Physicians and
  Surgeons
630 West 168th Street
New York, NY 10032
(212) 305–6905

Roswell Park Cancer Institute
Elm and Carlton Streets
Buffalo, NY 14263
(716) 845–4400

**Albert Einstein College of
Medicine**
1300 Morris Park Avenue
Bronx, NY 10461
(212) 920–4826

Kaplan Cancer Center
New York University Medical
  Center
462 First Avenue
New York, NY 10016-9103
(212) 263–6485

**University of Rochester Cancer
Center**
601 Elmwood Avenue, Box
  704
Rochester, NY 14642
(716) 275–4911

**NORTH CAROLINA
Duke Comprehensive Cancer
Center**
P.O. Box 3814
Durham, NC 27710
(919) 286–5515

**Lineberger Comprehensive
Cancer Center**
University of North Carolina
  Department of Medicine
Chapel Hill, NC 27599
(919) 966–4431

**Cancer Center of Wake Forest
University at the Bowman
Gray School of Medicine**
Medical Center Boulevard
Winston-Salem, NC 27157-1082
(919) 748–4354

**OHIO
Ohio State University
Comprehensive Cancer
Center**
410 West 10th Avenue
Columbus, OH 43210
(614) 293–8619

**Case Western Reserve
University**
University Hospitals of Cleveland
Ireland Cancer Center
2074 Abington Road
Cleveland, OH 44106
(216) 844–5432

**PENNSYLVANIA
Fox Chase Cancer Center**
7701 Burholme Avenue
Philadelphia, PA 19111
(215) 728–2570

**University of Pennsylvania
Cancer Center**
3400 Spruce Street
6th Fl. Penn Tower Hotel
Philadelphia, PA 19104
(215) 662–6364

Pittsburgh Cancer Institute
200 Meyran Avenue
Pittsburgh, PA 15213-2592
1–800–537–4063

**RHODE ISLAND
Roger Williams Cancer Center**
825 Chalkstone Avenue
Providence, RI 02908
(401) 456–2071

RESOURCES

TENNESSEE
Drew-Meharry-Morehouse
Consortium Cancer Center
1005 D.B. Todd Boulevard
Nashville, TN 37208
(615) 327–6927

St. Jude Children's Research
Hospital
332 North Lauderdale Street
Memphis, TN 38101-0318
(901) 522–0306

TEXAS
Institute for Cancer Research
and Care
4450 Medical Drive
San Antonio, TX 78229
(512) 616–5580

The University of Texas M. D.
Anderson Cancer Center
1515 Holcombe Boulevard
Houston, TX 77030
(713) 792–3245

UTAH
Utah Regional Cancer Center
University of Utah Medical
    Center
50 North Medical Drive, Room
    2C10
Salt Lake City, UT 84132
(801) 581–5052

VERMONT
Vermont Cancer Center
University of Vermont
1 South Prospect Street
Burlington, VT 05401
(802) 656–4580

VIRGINIA
Massey Cancer Center
Medical College of Virginia
Virginia Commonwealth
    University
1200 East Broad Street
Richmond, VA 23298
(804) 786–9641

WASHINGTON
Fred Hutchinson Cancer
Research Center
1124 Columbia Street
Seattle, WA 98104
(206) 467–4675

WISCONSIN
Wisconsin Clinical Cancer
Center
University of Wisconsin
600 Highland Avenue
Madison, WI 53792
(608) 263–8090

For additional information about cancer, write to the Office of Cancer Communications, National Cancer Institute, Bethesda, MD 20892, or call the toll-free telephone number of the Cancer Information Service at 1-800-4-CANCER. Spanish-speaking staff members are available.

AMERICAN CANCER SOCIETY, INC. CHARTERED DIVISIONS

Alabama Division, Inc.
504 Brookwood Boulevard
Homewood, Alabama 35209
(205) 879–2242

Alaska Division, Inc.
406 West Fireweed Lane
Suite 204
Anchorage, Alaska 99503
(907) 277–8696

Arizona Division, Inc.
2929 East Thomas Road
Phoenix, Arizona 85016
(602) 224–0524

Arkansas Division, Inc.
901 North University
Little Rock, Arkansas 72207
(501) 664–3480

California Division, Inc.
1710 Webster Street
P.O. Box 2061
Oakland, California 94612
(415) 893–7900

Colorado Division, Inc.
2255 South Oneida
P.O. Box 24669
Denver, Colorado 80224
(303) 758–2030

Connecticut Division, Inc.
Barnes Park South
14 Village Lane
Wallingford, Connecticut
  06492
(203) 265–7161

Delaware Division, Inc.
92 Read's Way, Suite 205
New Castle, Delaware 19720
(302) 324–4227

District of Columbia Division, Inc.
1875 Connecticut Avenue, NW
Suite 730
Washington, DC 20009
(202) 483–2600

Florida Division, Inc.
3709 West Jetton Avenue
Tampa, Florida 33629-5146
(813) 253–0541

Georgia Division, Inc.
Lenox Park
2200 Lake Boulevard
Atlanta, Georgia 30319
(404) 816–7800

Hawaii/Pacific Division, Inc.
Community Services Center Bldg.
200 North Vineyard Boulevard
Suite 100-A
Honolulu, Hawaii 96817
(808) 531–1662

Idaho Division, Inc.
2676 Vista Avenue
P.O. Box 5386
Boise, Idaho 83705
(208) 343–4609

Illinois Division, Inc.
77 East Monroe
Chicago, Illinois 60603
(312) 641–6150

Indiana Division, Inc.
8730 Commerce Park Place
Indianapolis, Indiana 46268
(317) 872–4432

Iowa Division, Inc.
8364 Hickman Road
Suite D
Des Moines, Iowa 50322
(515) 253–0147

Kansas Division, Inc.
1315 SW Arrowhead Road
Topeka, Kansas 66604-4020
(913) 273–4114

Kentucky Division, Inc.
701 West Muhammad Ali Blvd.
P.O. Box 1807
Louisville, Kentucky
  40201-1909
(502) 584–6782

Louisiana Division, Inc.
2200 Veterans Memorial
  Boulevard
Suite 214
Kenner, LA 70062
(504) 469–0021

Maine Division, Inc.
52 Federal Street
Brunswick, Maine 04011
(207) 729–3339

Maryland Division, Inc.
8219 Town Center Drive
Baltimore, Maryland
  21236-0026
(410) 931–6850

Massachusetts Division, Inc.
30 Speen Street
Framingham, Massachusetts
  01701-1800
(508) 270–4600

Michigan Division, Inc.
1205 East Saginaw Street
Lansing, Michigan 48906
(517) 371–2920

Minnesota Division, Inc.
3316 West 66th Street
Minneapolis, Minnesota 55435
(612) 925–2772

Mississippi Division, Inc.
1380 Livingston Lane
Lakeover Office Park
Jackson, Mississippi 39213
(601) 362–8874

Missouri Division, Inc.
3322 American Avenue
Jefferson City, Missouri 65102
(314) 893–4800

Montana Division, Inc.
17 North 26th Street
Billings, Montana 59101
(406) 252–7111

Nebraska Division, Inc.
8502 West Center Road
Omaha, Nebraska 68124-5255
(402) 393–5800

Nevada Division, Inc.
1325 East Harmon
Las Vegas, Nevada 89119
(702) 798–6857

New Hampshire Division, Inc.
Gail Singer Memorial Building
360 Route 101, Unit 501
Bedford, New Hampshire
  03110-5032
(603) 472–8899

New Jersey Division, Inc.
2600 US Highway 1
North Brunswick, New Jersey
  08902-6001
(201) 297–8000

New Mexico Division, Inc.
5800 Lomas Blvd., NE
Albuquerque, New Mexico
  87110
(505) 260–2105

New York State Division, Inc.
6725 Lyons Street
P.O. Box 7
East Syracuse, New York 13057
(315) 437–7025

Long Island Division, Inc.
75 Davids Drive
Hauppauge, New York 11788
(516) 436–7070

New York City Division, Inc.
19 West 56th Street
New York, New York 10019
(212) 586–8700

Queens Division, Inc.
112–25 Queens Boulevard
Forest Hills, New York
  11375
(718) 263–2224

Westchester Division, Inc.
30 Glenn Street
White Plains, New York
  10603
(914) 949–4800

North Carolina Division, Inc.
11 South Boylan Avenue
Suite 221
Raleigh, North Carolina 27603
(919) 834–8463

North Dakota Division, Inc.
1005 Westrac Drive
P.O. Box 426
Fargo, North Dakota 58103
(701) 232–1385

Ohio Division, Inc.
5555 Frantz Road
Dublin, Ohio 43017
(614) 889–9565

Oklahoma Division, Inc.
4323 NW 63rd
Suite 110
Oklahoma City, Oklahoma
  73112
(405) 843–9888

Oregon Division, Inc.
0330 SW Curry Street
Portland, Oregon 97201
(503) 295–6422

Pennsylvania Division, Inc.
P.O. Box 897
Route 422 & Sipe Avenue
Hershey, Pennsylvania
  17033-0897
(717) 533–6144

Philadelphia Division, Inc.
1626 Locust Street
Philadelphia, Pennsylvania
  19103
(215) 985–5400

Puerto Rico Division, Inc.
Calle Alverio #577
Esquina Sargento Medina
Hato Rey, Puerto Rico 00918
(809) 764–2295

Rhode Island Division, Inc.
400 Main Street
Pawtucket, Rhode Island
  02860
(401) 722–8480

South Carolina Division, Inc.
128 Stonemark Lane
Columbia, South Carolina
  29210-3855
(803) 750–1693

South Dakota Division, Inc.
4101 South Carnegie Place
Sioux Falls, South Dakota
  57106-2322
(605) 361–8277

Tennessee Division, Inc.
1315 Eighth Avenue, South
Nashville, Tennessee 37203
(615) 255–1227

Texas Division, Inc.
2433 Ridgepoint Drive
Austin, Texas 78754
(512) 928–2262

Utah Division, Inc.
941 East 3300 South
Salt Lake City, Utah 84106
(801) 483–1500

Vermont Division, Inc.
13 Loomis Street
Montpelier, Vermont 05602
(802) 223–2348

Virginia Division, Inc.
4240 Park Place Court
Glen Allen, Virginia 23060
(804) 527–3700

Washington Division, Inc.
2120 First Avenue North
Seattle, Washington
  98109-1140
(206) 283–1152

West Virginia Division, Inc.
2428 Kanawha Boulevard East
Charleston, West Virginia
  25311
(304) 344–3611

Wisconsin Division, Inc.
N19 W24350 Riverwood Drive
Waukesha, WI 53188
(414) 523–5500

Wyoming Division, Inc.
4202 Ridge Road
Cheyenne, Wyoming 82001
(307) 638–3331

Women with breast cancer who have concerns or questions about their workplace situation, insurance, or legal rights can request a free booklet, *Cancer: Your Job, Insurance and the Law,* by calling the American Cancer Society hotline at 1-800-ACS-2345.

NABCO BREAST CANCER RESOURCE LIST*

Regional Breast Cancer Support Groups
(alphabetical order by city/state)

Anchorage,	AK	The Anchorage Women's Breast Cancer Support Group (907) 261–3607
Gadsden,	AL	Woman to Woman (205) 543–8896
Tuscaloosa,	AL	UPFRONT Support Group (205) 759–7000
Fayetteville,	AR	Northwest Arkansas Cancer Support Home (501) 521–8024
Fort Smith,	AR	Phillips Cancer Support House (501) 782–6302
Little Rock,	AR	CARTI CancerAnswers (501) 664–8573
Phoenix,	AZ	Bosom Buddies (602) 231–6648
Phoenix,	AZ	Maryvale Samaritan Hospital (602) 848–5588
Scottsdale,	AZ	Y-ME Breast Cancer Network of Arizona (602) 231–6666
Tucson,	AZ	Arizona Cancer Center (520) 626–6044
Tucson,	AZ	Cerelle Center for Women's Health Breast Cancer Resource Center (602) 325–3000
Anaheim,	CA	Anaheim Memorial Hospital (714) 999–3880
Berkeley,	CA	Alta Bates (510) 204–1591
Berkeley,	CA	Woman's Cancer Resource Center (510) 548–9272
Chico,	CA	Beyond Breast Cancer Support Group (916) 892–6888
Encino,	CA	Vital Options (young adults) (818) 986–6368 fax
Escondido,	CA	Pallmar Pomerado Health System (619) 737–3960

* Copyright © 1995, National Alliance of Breast Cancer Organizations (NABCO), New York, NY. Excerpted and reprinted with permission.

Fresno,	CA	St. Agnes Medical Center (209) 449–5222
La Habra,	CA	Bloomers - Y-ME of Orange County (714) 447–6975
La Jolla,	CA	Scripps Memorial Hospital (619) 457–6756
La Jolla,	CA	UCSD Cancer Center (619) 543–6650
Lancaster,	CA	Ladies of Courage/Y-ME (805) 266–4811
Long Beach,	CA	Long Beach Memorial Breast Center (310) 933–7880
Long Beach,	CA	Y-ME South Bay/Long Beach (310) 984–8456
Lynwood,	CA	Sisters Network for African-American Women (310) 639–6511
Monterey,	CA	Breast Self-Help Group (408) 649–1772
Napa,	CA	Bosom Buddies (707) 257–4047
Orange,	CA	The Breast Care Center (714) 541–0101
Palm Springs,	CA	The Desert Comprehensive Breast Center (619) 323–6676
Palo Alto,	CA	Community Breast Health Project (415) 725–1788
Palo Alto,	CA	Discovery Breast Cancer Support Group/YWCA (415) 494–0972
Pasadena,	CA	Breast Cancer Networking Group (818) 796–1083
Sacramento,	CA	Save Ourselves/Y-ME of Sacramento (916) 921–9747
San Diego,	CA	Women's Cancer Task Force/Y-ME San Diego Chapter (619) 239–9283
San Francisco,	CA	Bay Area Lymphedema Support Group (415) 921–2911
San Francisco,	CA	Breast Cancer Action (415) 922–8279
San Francisco,	CA	The Breast Care Center (415) 476–5555

San Francisco,	CA	The Cancer Support Community (415) 648–9400
San Jose,	CA	Bay Area Breast Cancer Network (408) 261–1425
Santa Ana,	CA	Orange County Chapter Susan G. Komen Foundation (714) 480–5222
Santa Monica,	CA	Wellness Community (310) 314–2555
Sausalito,	CA	Center for Attitudinal Healing (415) 331–6161
Van Nuys,	CA	The Breast Center (818) 787–9911
Walnut Creek,	CA	John Muir Medical Center (510) 947–3322
West Covina,	CA	Queen of the Valley (818) 814–2464
Burlington, Ont.	CAN	Burlington Breast Cancer Support Services (905) 634–2333
St. Cath., Ont.	CAN	Breast Cancer Research and Education Fund (905) 687–3333
Col. Springs	CO	Penrose Cancer Center (719) 776–5273
Denver,	CO	AMC Cancer Research Center (303) 239–3424
Denver,	CO	Rose Breast Center (303) 320–7142
Denver,	CO	Rose Breast Center—Men's Discussion Group for Male Partners (303) 320–7142
Branford,	CT	Y-ME of New England (203) 483–8200
Danbury,	CT	I Can (203) 830–4621
Hartford,	CT	St. Francis Hospital and Medical Center (203) 548–4366
Norwalk,	CT	Cancer Care, Inc. (203) 854–9911
Ridgefield,	CT	Ridgefield Breast Cancer Support Group— The Revivers (203) 438–5555

Stamford,	CT	Building Bridges (203) 325–7447
Washington,	DC	Betty Ford Comprehensive Breast Center (202) 293–6654
Washington,	DC	George Washington University (202) 994–4589
Washington,	DC	Georgetown University (202) 784–4000
Washington,	DC	The Mary-Helen Mautner Project for Lesbians with Cancer (202) 332–5536
Wilmington,	DE	Looking Ahead Support Group (302) 421–4161
Coral Springs,	FL	Y-ME of Florida (305) 752–2101
Daytona Beach,	FL	Halifax Medical Center Women's Services (904) 254–4211
Jacksonville,	FL	Bosom Buddies (904) 633–8246
Miami,	FL	South Florida Comp. Cancer Center (305) 227–5582
Orlando,	FL	Center for Women's Medicine—Florida Hospital (407) 897–1617
Orlando,	FL	Bosom Buddies (407) 281–8663
Pensacola,	FL	Ann L. Baroco Center for Women's Health (904) 474–7878
Sarasota,	FL	Sarasota Memorial Hospital (813) 917–1375
Tampa,	FL	FACTORS / H. Lee Moffit Cancer Center (813) 972–8407
Atlanta,	GA	Northside Hospital (404) 851–8635
Tucker,	GA	Bosom Buddies of GA—also offers bone- marrow transplant support group (404) 493–7517
Tucker,	GA	Bosom Buddies of GA—Men's Bereavement Support Group (404) 493–7517
Honolulu,	HI	Queens Medical Center—Women of Spirit (808) 537–7555

Cedar Rapids,	IA	"ESPECIALLY FOR YOU" After Breast Cancer (800) 642–6329
Marshalltown,	IA	Marshalltown Support Group (515) 752–8775
Sioux City,	IA	ABC-After Breast Cancer Support Group (712) 279–2989
Waterloo,	IA	Breast Cancer Support Group (319) 292–2100
Boise,	ID	Mountain States Tumor Institute (208) 386–2764
Ketchum,	ID	The Wellness Group Hospice of the Wood River Valley (208) 726–8464
Alton,	IL	CARE—Alton Memorial Hospital (618) 463–7150
Barrington,	IL	Good Shepard Hospital (708) 381–9600, ext. 5336
Belleville,	IL	St. Elizabeth Hospital Mastectomy Club (618) 234–2120, ext. 1293
Chicago,	IL	Y-ME National Breast Cancer Organization (312) 986–8338
Decatur,	IL	Decatur Memorial Hospital (217) 876–2383
Elmhurst,	IL	Elmhurst Memorial Hospital (708) 833–1400, ext. 0111
Joliet,	IL	St. Joseph Medical Center (815) 741–7560
Macomb,	IL	McDonough District Hospital Women's Health Resource Center (309) 836–1584
Moline,	IL	Quad City Mastectomy Support Group (309) 764–2888
Pekin,	IL	Pekin Hospital—Mastectomy Support Group (309) 353–0807
Peoria,	IL	Susan G. Komen Breast Center (309) 689–6622
Rockford,	IL	Breast Cancer Support Group for Younger Women (815) 961–6215
Springfield,	IL	Sangamon Breast Cancer Support Group (217) 787–7187

Bluffton,	IN	Women's Cancer Support Group (219) 824–6493
Gary,	IN	Methodist Hospital (219) 886–4328
Indianapolis,	IN	Uplifter's Breast Cancer Support Group (317) 355–1411
Indianapolis,	IN	Y-ME of Central Indiana (317) 240–3331
Terre Haute,	IN	Y-ME of Wabash Valley (812) 877–3025
Warsaw,	IN	Women Winning Against Cancer (219) 269–9911
Wichita,	KS	Breast Cancer Care Group/Victory in the Valley (316) 262–7559
Ashland,	KY	Breast Cancer Support Group (606) 327–4535
Edgewood,	KY	St. Elizabeth Women's Center (606) 344–3939
Lexington,	KY	The Thursday Group (606) 269–4836
Owensboro,	KY	Women of Owensboro Mastectomy Association (800) 227–2345
Prestonsburg,	KY	Breast Cancer Support Group (606) 886–8511, ext. 7575
Marrero,	LA	Bosom Buddies—West Jefferson Medical Center (504) 349–1640
Metairie,	LA	Center For Living With Cancer (504) 454–4500
New Orleans,	LA	Breast Cancer Support Group (504) 897–4223
New Orleans,	LA	Ochsner Breast Cancer Support Group (504) 842–4251
New Orleans,	LA	Patricia Trost Friedler Cancer Counseling (504) 587–2120
Slidell,	LA	Bosom Buddies—NorthShore Regional Medical Center (504) 646–5014
Amherst,	MA	Margaret Gozlin Counseling Center (413) 256–4600

Boston,	MA	New England Medical Center (617) 636–9227
Boston,	MA	Dana Farber Cancer Institute (617) 632–3459
Boston,	MA	Faulkner Breast Centre Support Group (617) 983–7967
Burlington,	MA	Lahey Clinic Breast Cancer Treatment Center (617) 273–8989
Cambridge,	MA	Harvard University (617) 495–2936
Framingham,	MA	Metro West Medical Center (508) 383–1378
Marion,	MA	Strength for Tomorrow (508) 748–0561
Pittsfield,	MA	Y-ME of the Berkshires (413) 499–2486
Springfield,	MA	Comprehensive Breast Program at Baystate Medical Center (413) 784–8010
Worcester,	MA	U. of Mass. Breast Cancer Education Awareness Group (508) 856–3112
Hagerstown,	MD	Y-ME of the Cumberland Valley (301) 791–5843
Pasedena,	MD	Cancer Resource and Support Center (410) 760–CARE
Timonium,	MD	Arm In Arm (410) 494–0083
Ann Arbor,	MI	University Hospital (313) 936–9425
Capac,	MI	Breast Cancer Support Group (810) 395–7626
Detroit,	MI	Breast Cancer Support Group (313) 343–3684
Detroit,	MI	Comprehensive Breast Center—Harper Hospital (313) 745–2754
Detroit,	MI	Michigan Cancer Foundation—Breast Cancer Detection Center (313) 833–7700
E. Grand Rapids,	MI	"EXPRESSIONS" for Women (616) 957–3223

RESOURCES

Farmington Hills,	MI	Berry Health Center (313) 493–6507
Flint,	MI	McLaren Mastectomy Support Group (810) 762–2375
Grand Rapids,	MI	Woman to Woman—St. Mary's Breast Center (616) 774–6756
Lansing,	MI	WINS Support Group—Sparrow Regional Cancer Center (517) 483–2689
Marquette,	MI	Marquette General Hospital (906) 225–3500
Midland,	MI	Midland Community Cancer Services (517) 835–4841
Petoskey,	MI	Just for Us (616) 347–8443
Rockwood,	MI	"Unique" Breast Cancer Support Group (313) 833–0710, ext. 770
Duluth,	MN	Duluth Clinic—Breast Diagnostic Center (218) 725–3195
Fridley,	MN	Mercy Unity Oncology Services (612) 780–7780
St. Louis Park,	MN	Methodist Hospital (612) 932–6086
Kansas City,	MO	Cancer Hotline (816) 932–8453
Kansas City,	MO	Menorah Medical Center TOUCH Breast Cancer Program (816) 276–8848
Kansas City,	MO	The Cancer Institute of Health Midwest (816) 751–2929
Springfield,	MO	Mid-America Cancer Center—Breast Cancer Network (St. John's) (800) 432–CARE
Springfield,	MO	Reach Together (417) 886–LADY
St. Charles,	MO	St. Joseph Health Center (314) 947–5614
St. Louis,	MO	Barnes Jewish Hospital (314) 362–5574
St. Louis,	MO	St. Luke's Hospital (314) 851–6090

308

St. Louis,	MO	SHARE Breast Cancer Education and Support Center (314) 991–4424
St. Louis,	MO	St. John's Mercy Cancer Center (314) 569–6400
St. Louis,	MO	Missouri Baptist Medical Center (314) 569–5263
St. Louis,	MO	Young Mothers with Breast Cancer— Jewish Hospital CIRCLE (314) 454–8671
Biloxi,	MS	Biloxi Regional Medical Center (601) 436–1694
Sidney,	MT	Bosom Buddies (406) 482–2423
Asheville,	NC	Life After Cancer/Pathways, Inc. (704) 252–4106
Chapel Hill,	NC	Chapel Hill Support Group (919) 929–7022
Charlotte,	NC	Presbyterian Hospital (704) 384–4750
Charlotte,	NC	Women Living with Cancer (704) 355–2884
Durham,	NC	Duke Comprehensive Cancer Center (919) 684–4497
Raleigh,	NC	Triangle Breast Cancer Support Group (919) 881–9754
Rocky Mount,	NC	Boice Willis Clinic (919) 937–0200
Rocky Mount,	NC	Nash Day Hospital (919) 443–8607
Wilson,	NC	Kathy Farris Memorial Mastectomy Group (919) 237–0439
Winston-Salem,	NC	Pink Broomstick—Cancer Services, Inc. (910) 725–7421
Bismarck,	ND	Great Plains Rehabilitation Services— Mastectomy Support Group (701) 224–7988
Lincoln,	NE	St. Elizabeth Community Health Center (402) 486–7567
Concord,	NH	Breast Cancer Support Group (603) 224–2051
Concord,	NH	Concord Hospital (603) 225–2711, ext. 3053

Lebanon,	NH	Norris Cotton Cancer Center (603) 650–5789
Manchester,	NH	Catholic Medical Center (603) 626–2049
Manchester,	NH	Elliot Hospital (603) 628–2338
Bayonne,	NJ	Bayonne Hospital (201) 339–7573
Bergen County,	NJ	After Breast Cancer (201) 487–2224
Brick,	NJ	Brick Hospital (908) 295–6427
Bricktown,	NJ	Breast Disease & Surgery Center (908) 458–4600
Camden,	NJ	Cooper Hospital University Medical Center (609) 342–2474
Dover,	NJ	Northwest Covenant Health Care System (201) 989–3106
Fair Haven,	NJ	Mid Monmouth County Recurrence Support Group (908) 229–9535
Flemington,	NJ	Breast Cancer Support Group (908) 782–6112
Freehold,	NJ	Women's Health Center (908) 308–0292
Hackensack,	NJ	Hackensack Medical Center (201) 996–5800
Hunterdon,	NJ	Hunterdon Medical Center (908) 782–6112
Livingston,	NJ	St.Barnabas Medical Center (201) 533–8414
Long Branch,	NJ	Monmouth Medical Center (908) 870–5360
Millburn,	NJ	Cancer Care, Inc. (201) 379–7500
Neptune,	NJ	Jersey Shore Medical Center (908) 776–4240
New Brunswick,	NJ	Cancer Institute of New Jersey (908) 235–6790
Pomona,	NJ	Atlantic City Medical Center (609) 652–3500
Princeton,	NJ	Beyond Cancer (609) 683–0692

Princeton,	NJ	Breast Cancer Resource Center (for men and women)—Princeton YWCA (609) 497–2126
Randolf,	NJ	Women At Risk (for women considering prophylactic mastectomies) (800) 82–BREAST
Red Bank,	NJ	Riverview Regional Cancer Center (908) 530–2382
Ridgewood,	NJ	Cancer Care, Inc. (201) 444–6630
Ridgewood,	NJ	Valley Hospital (201) 447–8656
Somerville,	NJ	Somerset Medical Center (908) 685–2953
South River,	NJ	WISE—Women's International Support Environment (908) 257–6611
Summit,	NJ	Pathways (908) 277–3663
Toms River,	NJ	Community Medical Center (908) 240–8148
Wash. Township,	NJ	After Breast Cancer Surgery (201) 666–6610
Westfield,	NJ	CHEMOcare (800) 55–CHEMO / (908) 233–1103
Albuquerque,	NM	People Living Through Cancer (505) 242–3263
Farmington,	NM	The Four Corners Breast Cancer Support Group (505) 326–0743
Reno,	NV	St. Mary's Regional Medical Center (702) 789–3282
Binghamton,	NY	Brass Ears—Breast Cancer Support Group (607) 693–1759
Binghamton,	NY	Southern Tier Y-ME (607) 722–5839
Brooklyn,	NY	Cancer Institute of Brooklyn (718) 972–5816
Brooklyn,	NY	Long Island College Hospital (718) 780–2947
Buffalo,	NY	Breast Cancer Network of Western New York (716) 845–8086

Elmhurst,	NY	St. John's Queens Hospital (718) 457–1300, ext. 2250
Flushing,	NY	Flushing Hospital Medical Center (718) 670–5640
Garden City,	NY	Adelphi New York Statewide Breast Cancer HOTLINE and Support Program (516) 877–4444
Garden City,	NY	Sisters Network for African-American Women (516) 538–8086
Glens Falls,	NY	Glens Falls Hospital (518) 696–2000
Huntington,	NY	Huntington Hospital (516) 351–2568
Ithaca,	NY	Ithaca Breast Cancer Alliance (607) 277–9410
Ithaca,	NY	Tompkins Community Hospital (607) 274–4101
Johnson City,	NY	Women's Health Connection—United Health Services (607) 763–6546
Kingston,	NY	Benedictine Hospital (914) 334–3090
Manhasset,	NY	North Shore University Hospital (516) 926–HELP
New Hyde Park,	NY	Long Island Jewish Medical Center Post Lumpectomy Support Group (718) 470–7188
New York,	NY	Beth Israel Medical Center (212) 420–4230
New York,	NY	Beth Israel Medical Center (North Division) (212) 870–9502
New York,	NY	Breast Examination Center of Harlem (212) 864–0600
New York,	NY	Breast Friends—Mount Sinai Medical Center (212) 987–3063
New York,	NY	Cancer Care, Inc. (212) 302–2400
New York,	NY	Memorial Sloan-Kettering Cancer Center (212) 639–3292

New York,	NY	SHARE: Support Services for Women with Breast or Ovarian Cancer (212) 719–0364 / (212) 719–4454 (Spanish)
North Tarrytown,	NY	Side by Side (914) 347–2649
Pt. Jefferson,	NY	John T. Mather Memorial Hospital Live Love & Laugh Again (516) 476–2723
Putnam Valley,	NY	Breast Cancer Support Group (914) 528–8213
Rochester,	NY	Cancer Action Inc. (716) 423–9700
Rye Brook,	NY	Cancer Support Team, Inc. (914) 253–5334
Syosset,	NY	FEGS/Jewish Community Services (516) 364–8040
Valley Stream,	NY	Franklin Hospital (516) 256–6012
Woodbury,	NY	Cancer Care, Inc. (516) 364–8130
Cincinnati,	OH	Bethesda Oak Hospital Breast Center (513) 569–5152
Cincinnati,	OH	Cancer Family Care (513) 731–3346
Cincinnati,	OH	University of Cincinnati Hospital (513) 558–8567
Cleveland,	OH	Cleveland Clinic Foundation (216) 444–3770
Columbus,	OH	Arthur G. James Cancer Hospital (614) 293–3237
Columbus,	OH	Riverside Cancer Institute (614) 566–4321
Dayton,	OH	St. Elizabeth Breast Cancer (513) 229–7474
Dayton,	OH	Y-ME of the Greater Dayton Area (513) 274–9151
Hamilton,	OH	Fort Hamilton Hughes Hospital (513) 867–2700
Kettering,	OH	SOAR / Strength, Optimism & Recovery (513) 296–7231

Marietta,	OH	Marietta Memorial Hospital (614) 374–1450
Springfield,	OH	Mercy Medical Center (513) 390–5030
Youngstown,	OH	Southside Medical Center (216) 740–4176
Oklahoma City,	OK	Central Oklahoma Cancer Center (405) 636–7104
Oklahoma City,	OK	University of Oklahoma (405) 271–4514
Portland,	OR	St. Vincent Hospital (503) 291–4673
Springfield,	OR	McKenzie-Willamette Hospital (503) 726–4452
Tualatin,	OR	Meridian Park Hospital (503) 692–2113
Allentown,	PA	John and Dorothy Morgan Cancer Center (610) 402–0500
Bristol,	PA	Lower Bucks Hospital (215) 785–9056
Bryn Mawr,	PA	Bryn Mawr Hospital (610) 526–3073
Coatesville,	PA	Brandywine ABC Support Group (610) 383–8549
Dresher,	PA	Abington Memorial Hospital (215) 646–4954
Ft. Washington,	PA	Advanced Care Associates (800) 289–8001
Hershey,	PA	Milton S. Hershey Medical Center (717) 531–5867
Kingston,	PA	Wyoming Valley Health Care System (717) 283–7851
Lancaster,	PA	Lancaster Breast Cancer Network (717) 393–7477
Murraysville,	PA	Marie's Place (412) 459–0270
Norristown,	PA	Montgomery Breast Cancer Support Program (610) 270–2703
Philadelphia,	PA	Fox Chase Cancer Center (215) 728–2668
Philadelphia,	PA	Linda Creed Breast Cancer Foundation (215) 955–4354

Philadelphia,	PA	Thomas Jefferson University Hospital (215) 955–8370
Pittsburgh,	PA	Burger King Cancer Caring Center (412) 622–1212
Pittsburgh,	PA	Magee-Womens Hospital (412) 641–1178
Ridley Park,	PA	Taylor Hospital (610) 522–0203
West Reading,	PA	Breast Cancer Support Services of Berks County (610) 478–1447
York,	PA	York Cancer Center (717) 741–8100
Providence,	RI	Breast Health (401) 751–6890
Providence,	RI	Hope Center for Life Enhancement (401) 454–0404
Providence,	RI	Roger Williams Medical Center (401) 456–2284
(Statewide)	RI	Breast Cancer Support Groups (401) 822–0095
Columbia,	SC	Bosom Buddies and Man to Man (803) 771–5244
Columbia,	SC	Breast Cancer Support Group (803) 434–3378
Florence,	SC	McLeod Resource Center (803) 667–2888
Greenville,	SC	Breast Cancer Support Group (803) 455–7591
Lexington,	SC	Supporting Sisters (803) 796–6009
Sioux Falls,	SD	After Breast Cancer Survivors' Program (605) 333–5244
Chattanooga,	TN	Y-ME of Chattanooga (615) 886–4171
Knoxville,	TN	Breast Cancer Networker (615) 546–4661
Knoxville,	TN	Knoxville Breast Center (615) 584–0291
Nashville,	TN	Mastectomy Support Group (615) 665–0628
Arlington,	TX	Together We Will (817) 277–7434

Dallas,	TX	Between US
		(214) 521–5225
Dallas,	TX	Common Cares
		(214) 692–8893
Dallas,	TX	Patient to Patient
		(214) 821–2962
Dallas	TX	Sisters Network for African-American Women
		(214) 699–5105
Dallas,	TX	Charles A. Sammons Cancer Center
		(214) 820–2608
Dallas,	TX	Presbyterian Hospital of Dallas
		(214) 345–2600
Dallas,	TX	Medical City Hospital
		(214) 562–7717
Fort Worth,	TX	Breast Reconstruction Educational Support Group
		(817) 335–6363
Fort Worth,	TX	Doris Kupferle Breast Center
		(817) 882–3650
Houston,	TX	Sisters Network for African-American Women
		(713) 781–0255
Houston,	TX	The Rose Garden
		(713) 484–4708
Houston,	TX	The Rosebuds
		(713) 665–2729
Lake Jackson,	TX	Sisters Network for African-American Women
		(409) 297–4419
Plano,	TX	North Texas Cancer Center
		(214) 867–3577
Richardson,	TX	Bosom Buddies
		(214) 238–9516
Salt Lake City,	UT	Salt Lake Regional Breast Care Center
		(801) 350–4973
Vernal,	UT	Ashley Valley Medical Center
		(801) 789–3342
Alexandria,	VA	My Image After Breast Cancer
		(703) 461–9616
Charlottesville,	VA	Martha Jefferson Hospital
		(804) 982–8407

Falls Church,	VA	Fairfax Hospital (703) 698–3731
Harrisonburg,	VA	Rockingham Memorial Hospital (703) 433–4641
Norfolk,	VA	Sentara Leigh Hospital (804) 466–6837
Norfolk,	VA	Sentara Norfolk General (804) 668–4268
Richmond,	VA	Massey Cancer Center (804) 828–0450
Salem,	VA	Lewis-Gale Regional Cancer Center (800) 543–5660
Burlington,	VT	Breast Care Center (802) 656–2262
Bellevue,	WA	Overlake Hospital (206) 688–5261
Bremerton,	WA	Breast Cancer Support Group of Kitsap Co. (360) 373–1057
Edmonds,	WA	Puget Sound Tumor Institute (206) 640–4300
Everett,	WA	Providence General Medical Center (206) 258–7255
Kirkland,	WA	Evergreen Hospital (206) 899–2265
Mount Vernon,	WA	North Puget Oncology (360) 428–2146
Olympia,	WA	St. Peter Hospital Regional Cancer Center (206) 493–7510
Port Ludlow,	WA	CANHELP, Inc. (treatment decisions) (206) 437–2291
Seattle,	WA	Highline Community Hospital (206) 439–5577
Seattle,	WA	Providence (206) 320–2100
Seattle,	WA	Northwest Hospital (206) 368–1457
Seattle,	WA	Swedish Hospital Tumor Institute (206) 386–2323
Madison,	WI	Meriter Hospital Women's Center (608) 258–3750
Sheboygan,	WI	Sheboygan Memorial Medical Center (414) 451–5536

Charleston,	WV	Women & Children's Hospital
		(304) 348–2545
Cheyenne,	WY	United Medical Center
		(307) 633–7532

CANADIAN SUPPORT AND INFORMATION SERVICES

Cancer Information Service
(905) 387–1153 or 1 (800) 263–6750

Information and answers to questions about treatment, research, and statistics

Canadian Cancer Society
 Hamilton, Ontario   (905) 527–4555
 Oakville, Ontario   (905) 845–5231
 Burlington, Ontario   (905) 332–0060

Transportation, support groups, Reach to Recovery volunteers, educational information

Burlington Breast Cancer Support Services, Inc.
Burlington, Ontario   (905) 634–2333

Self-help group for women living with breast cancer

Toronto Sunnybrook Cancer Center
2075 Bayview Avenue
North York, Ontario M4N 3M5
(416) 488–5801

National resource directory of goods and services for managing changes in appearance brought on by cancer treatment

Mission Air Transportation Network
77 Bloor Street, Suite 1711
Toronto, Ontario M5S 3A1
(416) 222–6335

Nationwide program to give patients with cancer the use of available seats on corporate aircraft to get to and from recognized treatment centers

Cancer Counseling Center
Toronto, Ontario
(416) 778–4567

Counseling for individuals, couples, or groups based on the Simonton method

INDEX

ABOUT THE AUTHORS

Yashar Hirshaut is a medical oncologist specializing in the treatment of breast cancer. A graduate of the Albert Einstein College of Medicine, he completed his oncology training at the National Cancer Institute in Bethesda, Maryland, and at the Memorial Sloan-Kettering Cancer Center in New York. From 1970 to 1986 he served as an attending physician at Memorial Sloan-Kettering on the Clinical Immunology Service and as associate professor of medicine at the Cornell University Medical College. He was also head of the Laboratory for Immunodiagnosis at Sloan-Kettering. In addition to being in private practice, he is currently adjunct professor of biology at Yeshiva University and an attending physician at the Beth Israel Medical Center and Lenox Hill Hospital in New York City. Dr. Hirshaut has been editor of the professional journal *Cancer Investigation* since 1981. He is president of the Israel Cancer Research Fund and of a biotechnology firm, ImmunoSciences, Inc., which specializes in cancer therapy.

Peter I. Pressman is a surgical oncologist who specializes in the treatment of breast cancer. A graduate of Columbia College and the Columbia University College of Physicians and Surgeons, he trained at Presbyterian Hospital and the Columbia Division of Bellevue Hospital in New York City. Dr. Pressman has been in private practice in New York for over twenty-five years. He is associate clinical professor of surgery at the Albert Einstein School of Medicine and attending surgeon at the Beth Israel Medical Center and Lenox Hill Hospital. He has been consultant to the Guttman Breast Diagnostic Institute and president of the New York Metropolitan Breast Cancer Group, as well as a member of the Board of Directors (New York City division) and the Breast Cancer Detection and Treatment Subcommittee (National) of the American Cancer Society. He has published widely in the medical literature and has been named by *American Health, Good Housekeeping, New York,* and *Town and Country* magazines as among the best breast cancer doctors in New York City and in the nation.